NATIONAL
ACADEMIES

Sciences
Engineering
Medicine

NATIONAL
ACADEMIES
PRESS
Washington, DC

Whole-Person Oral Health Education

Maartje Wouters and Patricia Cuff,
Rapporteurs

Global Forum on Innovation in
Health Professional Education

Board on Global Health

Health and Medicine Division

Proceedings of a Workshop

NATIONAL ACADEMIES PRESS 500 Fifth Street, NW Washington, DC 20001

This activity was supported by contracts between the National Academy of Sciences and Academy of Integrative Health and Medicine, Academy of Nutrition and Dietetics, Accreditation Council for Graduate Medical Education, American Academy of Nursing, American Association of Colleges of Osteopathic Medicine, American Board of Family Medicine, American Council of Academic Physical Therapy, American Dental Education Association, American Medical Association, American Nurses Credentialing Center, American Occupational Therapy Association, American Physical Therapy Association, American Psychological Association, American Speech-Language-Hearing Association, Association of American Medical Colleges, Association of Schools and Colleges of Optometry, Association of Schools of Advancing Health Professions, Athletic Training Strategic Alliance, Columbia University Vagelos College of Physicians and Surgeons, Council on Social Work Education, Massachusetts General Hospital Institute of Health Professions, National Academies of Practice, National Association of Social Workers, National Board for Certified Counselors and Affiliates, National Board of Medical Examiners, National Council of State Boards of Nursing, National League for Nursing, Physician Assistant Education Association, National Register of Health Service Psychologists, Society for Simulation in Healthcare, Texas Tech University Health Sciences Center, U.S. Department of Veterans Affairs, and Weill Cornell Medicine—Qatar. Any opinions, findings, conclusions, or recommendations expressed in this publication do not necessarily reflect the views of any organization or agency that provided support for the project.

International Standard Book Number-13: 978-0-309-71880-6
International Standard Book Number-10: 0-309-71880-5
Digital Object Identifier: https://doi.org/10.17226/27761

This publication is available from the National Academies Press, 500 Fifth Street, NW, Keck 360, Washington, DC 20001; (800) 624-6242 or (202) 334-3313; http://www.nap.edu.

Printed in the United States of America.

Suggested citation: National Academies of Sciences, Engineering, and Medicine. 2024. *Whole-person oral health education: Proceedings of a workshop*. The National Academies Press. https://doi.org/10.17226/27761.

The **National Academy of Sciences** was established in 1863 by an Act of Congress, signed by President Lincoln, as a private, nongovernmental institution to advise the nation on issues related to science and technology. Members are elected by their peers for outstanding contributions to research. Dr. Marcia McNutt is president.

The **National Academy of Engineering** was established in 1964 under the charter of the National Academy of Sciences to bring the practices of engineering to advising the nation. Members are elected by their peers for extraordinary contributions to engineering. Dr. John L. Anderson is president.

The **National Academy of Medicine** (formerly the Institute of Medicine) was established in 1970 under the charter of the National Academy of Sciences to advise the nation on medical and health issues. Members are elected by their peers for distinguished contributions to medicine and health. Dr. Victor J. Dzau is president.

The three Academies work together as the **National Academies of Sciences, Engineering, and Medicine** to provide independent, objective analysis and advice to the nation and conduct other activities to solve complex problems and inform public policy decisions. The National Academies also encourage education and research, recognize outstanding contributions to knowledge, and increase public understanding in matters of science, engineering, and medicine.

Learn more about the National Academies of Sciences, Engineering, and Medicine at **www.nationalacademies.org**.

PLANNING COMMITTEE ON SHARING MODELS OF WHOLE-PERSON ORAL HEALTH EDUCATION[1]

BRUCE DOLL (*Cochair*), Uniformed Services University of Health Sciences
ANITA GLICKEN (*Cochair*), University of Colorado Anschutz Medical Center
RICHARD BERMAN, University of South Florida
URSHLA DEVALIA, Royal National ENT and Eastman Dental Hospital, University College Hospital, London
KAREN HALL, Capitol Dental Care
DONNA HALLAS, New York University
JOHN KEMP, Lakeshore Foundation
CYNTHIA LORD, Lake County Free Clinic Ohio
CLEOPATRA MATANHIRE, University of Zimbabwe
TERESA MARSHALL, University of Iowa
DANIEL McNEIL, University of Florida
LEMMIETTA McNEILLY, American Speech-Language-Hearing Association
KUDZAI MUREMBWE-MACHINGAUTA, Africa University, Zimbabwe
JEFFERY STEWART, American Dental Education Association
RITA S. VILLENA, University San Martin de Porres
MARKO VUJICIC, Health Policy Institute
ROBERT WEYANT, University of Pittsburgh
MARK S. WOLFF, University of Pennsylvania, School of Dental Medicine

Consultants

JULIAN FISHER, University of Pennsylvania, School of Dental Medicine
ISABEL GARCIA, University of Florida, College of Dentistry
MICHAEL GLICK, University of Pennsylvania, School of Dental Medicine
ZOHRAY TALIB, California University of Science and Medicine

Staff

PATRICIA A. CUFF, Senior Program Officer
ERIKA CHOW, Research Assistant
JULIE PAVLIN, Senior Director, Board on Global Health

---

[1] The National Academies of Sciences, Engineering, and Medicine's forums and roundtables do not issue, review, or approve individual documents. The responsibility for the published Proceedings of a Workshop rests with the workshop rapporteurs and the institution.

Reviewers

This Proceedings of a Workshop was reviewed in draft form by individuals chosen for their diverse perspectives and technical expertise. The purpose of this independent review is to provide candid and critical comments that will assist the National Academies of Sciences, Engineering, and Medicine in making each published proceedings as sound as possible and to ensure that it meets the institutional standards for quality, objectivity, evidence, and responsiveness to the charge. The review comments and draft manuscript remain confidential to protect the integrity of the process.

We thank the following individuals for their review of this proceedings:

RICHARD BERMAN, University of South Florida
HELEN LEE, University of Illinois Chicago, College of Medicine
HUGH SILK, University of Massachusetts, Chan Medical School
JANE ZIEGLER, Rutgers, the State University of New Jersey

Although the reviewers listed above provided many constructive comments and suggestions, they were not asked to endorse the content of the proceedings nor did they see the final draft before its release. The review of this proceedings was overseen by **CASWELL EVANS,** University of Illinois Chicago, College of Dentistry. He was responsible for making certain that an independent examination of this proceedings was carried out in accordance with standards of the National Academies and that all review comments were carefully considered. Responsibility for the final content rests entirely with the rapporteurs and the National Academies.

Acknowledgments

The National Academies of Sciences, Engineering, and Medicine's Global Forum on Innovation in Health Professional Education wishes to express its sincere gratitude to Penn Dental Medicine who collaborated to co-host the workshop at the University of Pennsylvania in Philadelphia. Deep appreciation goes to staff at Penn Dental Medicine for their logistical support in the workshop process, especially Elizabeth Ketterlinus, Jennifer Pacitti, and Pamela Rice.

The forum wishes to thank all members of the planning committee, who collaborated to ensure a workshop replete with informative presentations and moderated rich discussions. The forum is grateful for the support of our workshop sponsors, without which we could not have undertaken this project. Finally, the forum thanks workshop speakers, who generously shared their subject-matter expertise and time with workshop participants.

Contents

1 Introduction 1

2 Framing the Workshop Objectives 7
VALUE OF ORAL HEALTH PROMOTION AND DISEASE
PREVENTION, 8
DIALOGUE WITH THE INTERPROFESSIONAL
PANELISTS, 16

3 Understanding the Value Proposition in Oral Health 21
VALUE PROPOSITION FOR ORAL HEALTH, 22
DEMONSTRATING THE VALUE PROPOSITION FOR
PERSONS WITH DISABILITIES, 31
VESTED INTEREST GROUP INPUT ON A POTENTIAL
VALUE PROPOSITION, 35

4 Whole Health Through Oral Health 45
SCHOOL-BASED HEALTH CENTERS, 46
ORAL HEALTH PROMOTION AND CARE FOR
PATIENTS WITH MENTAL HEALTH CONDITIONS
IN ZIMBABWE, 47
INTEGRATING ORAL HEALTH INTO GENERAL HEALTH
AT INFANCY, 48
COMMUNITY-BASED OUTREACH EDUCATION IN
FLORIDA, 49
MINI MOUTH CARE MATTERS IN ENGLAND, 49

5 **Fitting the Value Proposition into the Larger Picture**   53
   ORAL HEALTH EQUITY, 54
   A WHOLE ORAL HEALTH HOME, 57
   A VALUE PROPOSITION REVISITED, 61
   OPEN DISCUSSION, 62
   CLOSING, 67

APPENDIXES

A References   69
B Workshop Agenda   73
C Workshop Planning Committee Biographical Sketches   81
D Workshop Speaker Biographical Sketches   95
E Members of the Global Forum on Innovation in Health
   Professional Education   101

Boxes, Figures, and Tables

BOXES

1-1 Statement of Task, 2

2-1 Key Points Made by Individual Speakers, 7

3-1 Key Points Made by Individual Speakers, 21

4-1 Key Points Made by Individual Speakers, 45

5-1 Key Points Made by Individual Speakers, 53

FIGURES

3-1 The business model canvas, 23
3-2 The value proposition should solve pains and enhance gains for each vested interest group, 24
3-3 Where patients present with oral health needs, 29
3-4 Oral health value proposition for persons with disabilities, 37
3-5 Oral health value proposition for educators and providers, 41
3-6 Oral health value proposition for payers and policy makers, 43

5-1 The difference between equality, equity, and justice in health care, 54
5-2 A framework for the definition of oral health, 59
5-3 Value proposition word cloud, 62

TABLES

3-1   Oral Health Value Proposition Pains for Persons with Disabilities, 36
3-2   Oral Health Value Proposition Gains for Persons with Disabilities, 36
3-3a Oral Health Value Proposition Pains for Providers, 38
3-3b Oral Health Value Proposition Pains for Educators, 39
3-4   Oral Health Value Proposition Gains for Educators and Providers, 39
3-5   Oral Health Value Proposition Pains for Payers and Policy Makers, 42
3-6   Oral Health Value Proposition Gains for Payers and Policy Makers, 42

1

Introduction[1]

On February 15–16, 2024, the Global Forum on Innovation in Health Professional Education at the National Academies of Sciences, Engineering, and Medicine held a hybrid workshop at the University of Pennsylvania's Penn Dental Medicine that was designed to provide unique learning opportunities for exploring a value proposition for holistic oral health. The workshop engaged experts from around the globe representing multiple sectors and professions to learn from and with each other about best practices for providing interprofessional, compassionate, cost-effective oral health prevention and care for persons with disabilities. Workshop presenters defined disabilities broadly to include anyone with a physical or mental health challenge. This includes those who were born with a disability and those who acquired the disability at any stage of life from infancy through older ages, permanently or temporarily, and regardless of whether or not the person works in the health professions. The workshop was planned by an expert planning committee based on the statement of task of the workshop (see Box 1-1). Discussions at the workshop were universal in nature and were intended to contribute to the broader understanding of whole-person oral health education.

[1] The planning committee's role was limited to planning the workshop. This Proceedings of a Workshop was prepared by independent rapporteurs as a factual account of what occurred at the workshop. The statements, recommendations, and opinions expressed are those of individual presenters and participants and are not necessarily endorsed or verified by the National Academies of Sciences, Engineering, and Medicine. They should not be construed as reflecting any group consensus.

BOX 1-1
Statement of Task

A planning committee of the National Academies of Sciences, Engineering, and Medicine will organize and conduct a public workshop to learn from examples of interprofessional holistic oral health education from across the learning continuum. Invited presentations and discussions will involve global audiences in exploring a value proposition for educational models aimed at improving the health of underserved persons and communities through oral health promotion and prevention efforts. The UN Sustainable Development Goals could be a platform on which to discuss the value proposition.

Chapter 1 of these proceedings details the opening remarks and the objectives of the workshop. Chapter 2 lays out the presentations that frame the workshop objectives, focusing on the value of oral health, particularly for those with disabilities, and discusses the importance of interprofessional education and collaboration practice for a holistic approach to oral health promotion. Chapter 3 explores a value proposition for oral health promotion and disease prevention from multiple vested interest group perspectives and also includes the outcomes of breakout session discussions. Chapter 4 focuses on national and international examples of Whole Health through oral health, and Chapter 5 situates the value proposition within the larger community ecosystem by discussing oral health equity and the Whole Health home. Chapter 6 describes the closing session of the workshop that included a reflective roundtable discussion on lessons learned and final remarks on health equity that closed the workshop. Appendix A contains a list of references, and Appendix B contains the workshop agenda. Biographies of the Workshop Planning Committee and Speakers are provided in Appendix C and D, respectively. Lastly, members of the Global Forum on Innovation in Health Professional Education that hosted the workshop are listed in Appendix E.

Opening the workshop, Bruce Doll, from the Office of Research at Uniformed Services University, briefly summarized the different sessions of the workshop and emphasized that each attendee has perspectives and expectations that can complement the planned sessions to achieve the objectives of the workshop. He discussed his personal experiences in rural areas of Alaska, Thailand, the Philippines, and Haiti, where delivery of general and oral health care differed greatly from his other work experiences. In these rural communities, he worked with internists, nurses, public health professionals, and veterinarians, and they all had to find ways to work together to improve oral health. The challenging, constrained environment required adapting spontaneously to achieve favorable outcomes, and Doll found that planning for the unexpected was critical.

Doll noted that to maximize outcomes for all three of the vested interest groups—patients, providers, and payers—all three must embrace a commonly generated and collectively executed value proposition (described in Chapter 3). To achieve the desired outcome of oral health promotion and disease prevention, he noted, all three vested interest groups would have to work together. Drawing upon his past experiences as a rural dental provider with global experience made Doll realize that health promotion efforts must be approached with cultural humility and align with a community's deeply held beliefs, expectations, infrastructure, and a host of other factors. In oral health, he found that the spontaneity he and his colleagues were forced to employ fell short of what he believes is the highest goal—young people retaining their teeth. But for this to happen, Doll said, planning is key. He finished by emphasizing the importance of active participation by all the attendees to make the meeting meaningful for those in the room as well as for those joining virtually.

Following Doll, Anita Glicken, the executive director of the National Interprofessional Initiative on Oral Health, noted that every person looks through a different window when it comes to the perceived value of whole-person interprofessional oral health care. Glicken is also a clinical social worker, and she discussed what her work as a social worker has to do with oral health care, something that is not always well understood. Glicken mentioned that each profession has its own contribution to patient health, but only together can they serve the whole person; unfortunately, people often work within their silos in a fragmented health care system. In the United States, each year 109 million people see a physician but do not visit a dentist, while 29 million people visit a dentist but do not see a physician, she said. Glicken discussed how this fragmentation of care affects a provider's communication with a patient, as well as the flow of information between providers about their patient's health.

Currently, she said, there is little to no communication between dental providers and medical care professionals. In an example, she discussed how people with chronic illnesses, such as diabetes, are responsible for conveying medical information about their illness and medication use to their dentist and conversely, dental information to their medical health care team. According to Glicken, this is a serious burden on the patient and an unreliable way of communicating critical health information. Some other examples Glicken mentioned were the role oral pathogenic bacteria play in chronic diseases such as diabetes, and she also wondered how often it is considered how mental health might play a role in the care and progression of oral disease or the combination of chronic illnesses and mental health.

Glicken noted that access to care is another significant barrier: 58 million Americans are living in dental health professional shortage areas (HRSA, 2024), and 68.5 million adults are without dental insurance or dental coverage (CareQuest Institute for Oral Health, 2023). These people often end up in the emergency room (ER), resulting in 2 million ER visits for nontraumatic dental problems each year (Akinlotan and Ferdinand, 2020).

Poor oral health can often be prevented, Glicken remarked, so it is important to ask, who else in the workforce can be recruited to participate in prevention? A national interprofessional initiative was formed in 2009, the National Interprofessional Initiative on Oral Health (NIIOH), which is a consortium of payers, health professionals, and national organizations. NIIOH is a system change initiative that provides "backbone support" and facilitates interprofessional agreement and alignment to prepare an interprofessional oral health workforce for whole-person care. Given the critical relationship of oral health to overall health, said Glicken, through interprofessional collaborations NIIOH members are able to contribute to conversations in substantive ways about improving health equity and lowering costs. Their work follows the assumption that if oral health can be integrated into primary care education and professional coursework, providers would enter the workforce ready and willing to partner.

Glicken continued by explaining that all-health integration is not a new concept. In 2000, a surgeon general's report first called attention to the issues of disparity and access to care, and the oral–systemic connection that could potentially be addressed through an interprofessional shared collaborative approach to whole-person care (HHS, 2000). However, according to Glicken, the subsequent call to action was largely ignored until two documents gave a big lift to the oral health integration movement a decade later. The first was a report on the integration of oral health and primary care practice, describing what can be done by defining a set of oral health core clinical competencies for nondental providers (NIH, 2021). The second was the interprofessional education collaboratives core competencies for practice, which describe what can be done together through a comprehensive team-based care environment (IPEC, 2023). These challenges and strategies subsequently inspired a philosophy of collective impact where people work within and across health professions to create a movement that drives change using the unique capacities of each health professional to maximize the effect, Glicken said.

Today, thousands of health professions students and clinicians are learning to think differently about how to work together. Glicken remarked that Smiles for Life, a comprehensive and widely used national oral health curriculum, is free to access online and includes up to 8 hours of free continuing education. The site has been visited more than 3 million times, and over 500,000 courses have been completed for credit. Educators can download module content to use in education, so the real reach of the program is even broader, said Glicken. Eight health professions and over 20 professional organizations endorsed it, which helped the widespread use.

Glicken ended her talk by saying that during the workshop, participants would explore the concept of whole-person care. Doing so, she said, could improve access and value of care for persons with physical and mental disabilities by bridging professional silos and focusing on disease prevention, valued care, and population health through interprofessional oral health efforts.

2

Framing the Workshop Objectives

BOX 2-1
Key Points Made by Individual Speakers*

- Results showed that when reimbursements were improved, there was an increase in the use of preventive dentistry. (Lee)
- Providing preventive services in the community could reserve the dental office for complex treatments that can only be performed in that environment. (Glassman)
- Patients who are treated by a team of experts and specialists [in the hospital] are likely to receive a more holistic approach to their disease management, health, and recovery. (Hall)
- Nursing students can teach dental students how to take comprehensive patient histories, while dental students can teach nursing students how to manage and help patients during dental procedures. (Hallas)
- A student-managed health clinic brings teams of social work, physician assistants, medical nursing, and dental students together using a shared visit model. (Lord)
- Bringing the larger health community into a conversation can help spread the message that diet-related risk factors are the same for oral and systemic diseases, which can both be addressed as a team. (Marshall)
- Clinical health psychology can play a part in working together with other professions to change behavior at various levels, such as the behavior of providers, policy makers, and payers. (McNeil)

* This list is the rapporteurs' summary of points made by the individual speakers identified, and the statements have not been endorsed or verified by the National Academies of Sciences, Engineering, and Medicine. They are not intended to reflect a consensus among workshop participants.

VALUE OF ORAL HEALTH PROMOTION
AND DISEASE PREVENTION

The session moderator, Isabel Garcia, dean of University of Florida's College of Dentistry, opened by providing context for the workshop objectives. She discussed how the definition of oral health, as defined by bodies such as the FDI World Dental Federation (FDI, n.d.) and the World Health Organization (WHO, 2024), has shifted from the mere absence of disease to one that focuses on wellness and well-being. This shift, Garcia stated, makes it clear that oral health is a fundamental human right and should be part of health policies. Furthermore, calling oral health a human right provides the impetus for the oral health community to work with others outside of dentistry to reach the goal of oral health wellness and well-being. In recent years, she continued, there has been more recognition of the need to close the divide between dentistry and medicine that has contributed to inefficiency, dysfunction, and neglect of oral health. As dean of a dental school, Garcia believes that dental schools could contribute by adding more interprofessional and community-engaged education to their curricula and by expanding the interventions that reach out to the community. Garcia ended her introduction by emphasizing that this is a time for action as previous efforts in oral health have fallen short by not adequately addressing the oral health needs of underserved populations, particularly for people with special needs and disabilities.

The Value of Oral Health Promotion and Disease Prevention
to Limit the Need for Costly or Invasive Interventions

Helen H. Lee is an associate professor at the Department of Anesthesiology, College of Medicine, at the University of Illinois Chicago, and director of the Medical Scholars program. Her research and work as a pediatric anesthesiologist focuses on oral health. Lee discussed her journey in becoming interested in the topic after first observing who was receiving care in the emergency room to treat toothache pain. To investigate this, Lee and her colleagues performed a series of studies, which showed racial and ethnic disparities in who gets treated and receives opioids, and disparities in terms of socioeconomic factors (Lee et al., 2012, 2016; Lewis et al., 2015). She and her team then conducted a series of studies to better understand the children who come to the operating room (OR) and receive general anesthesia for dental treatments (Lee et al., 2019, 2020a,b,c). They assessed how use and surgical rates are being determined by state Medicaid programs and found tremendous variability by state in terms of providing access and setting funding priorities. Their research then focused on the question, if policy levers were moved to increase access to preventive care through Medicaid reimbursements to dentistry, would that have long-term oral health outcomes? Additionally, would this approach lead to fewer children in the OR for general anesthesia? Results showed that when reimbursements were improved, there was an increase in the use of preventive dentistry. However, it did not make a difference for OR use (Lee et al., 2020a). Next, Lee focused on a public health intervention, which was access to community water fluoridation (Lee, 2020c). This intervention also did not lead to differences in surgical service use. Based on the research, Lee inferred that disease would persist when using a single intervention that only targets one layer of the social determinants.

Lee then provided an overview of the research done by Bruen et al. (2016) on several Medicaid state programs. These data showed that very small proportions of the population represented high users and large expenditures on state Medicaid programs for severe disease. Up to 50 percent of children that present for general anesthesia with severe cavities will develop a cavity again within 6 to 12 months. The research by Bruen et al. calculated the estimated costs of dental care under general anesthesia at $450 million in 2011 (Bruen et al., 2016), but this did not address children presenting in dental offices receiving general anesthesia. Lee's research showed that in some states, a large proportion of general anesthesia cases were performed in dental offices, so the reported $450 million by Bruen et al. is likely an underestimation.

Additionally, even when high-risk populations—defined based on race/ethnicity or socioeconomic background—are provided access to regular preventive dental care, the disease persists (Lin et al., 2018). Therefore, Lee suggested there is a need to reflect more on what people do in their daily lives that keep them healthy, in particular, those who are at high risk. She then commented that this information is largely absent from the literature. Lee then acknowledged "some bumps with interprofessional collaboration" for things such as reimbursement and coding. While these are tied together, Lee sees each of them currently as obstacles to holistic care. It is very challenging to link the records between dentistry and medicine and, she added, funding and credit are issues multidisciplinary teams often grapple with.

The general public could benefit from more information on the importance of oral health promotion with disease prevention that is reinforced across multiple professions, she continued. Lee then noted that changes can be made to the future workforce by educating health professional learners when they are in school, but there is also potential to educate undergraduates before they decide which branch of health care they will specialize in. Reaching students early is when Lee believes learners are more open to the idea that the mouth is part of the body.

Lee closed with three examples of integrated health delivery systems. The first is out of the University of Illinois where interdisciplinary teams made up of medicine, dentistry, and psychology practitioners, community health workers, and hygienists work with community partners in medical and dental clinics to promote oral health and prevent chronic disease in children through prevention efforts (CO-OP Chicago, n.d.). The second, in North Carolina, involves a collaboration between medicine and dentistry focusing on prenatal oral health with the aim of having a multigenerational effect (PHOP, n.d.). The third is one that Lee herself is the coprincipal investigator. Known as PROTECT, this is a clinical trial looking at children presenting for anesthesia to manage severe dental disease, in which caregivers are provided with a parenting support program to promote health through healthy behaviors. PROTECT involves a collaboration among pediatric anesthesiology, clinical and community psychology, pediatrics, pediatric dentistry, and community health workers (University of Illinois Chicago College of Dentistry, 2024).

Oral Disease Prevention and Oral Health Promotion to Maximize Oral Health Care Experiences and Outcomes for Persons with Disabilities

Paul Glassman, the associate dean for research and community engagement at the College of Dental Medicine at California Northstate University, attended the meeting virtually. Glassman noted that a lot of money is paid for dental care. It is one of the most expensive sectors of health care in the United States, but the money is not spent effectively. He asked how oral health care can be better provided, in particular, for persons with disabilities. He described the situation for this population as "pretty dire." According to a report produced by the Sacramento County Department of Health (2022) in California, many people with disabilities, not just in California, go into dental offices but are told they cannot be seen there. This means that persons with disabilities have no other option but to undergo general anesthesia for dental treatments rather than receive preventive care as an outpatient in a dental or health care clinic. Glassman argued that often, the rush to treatment using anesthesia is made too quickly, sometimes resulting in waits of up to 4 years before receiving treatment (Glassman et al., 2009).

The emphasis in the U.S. health system on treating oral disease seems to be in the wrong place. As a result, money is spent incorrectly; expensive care is prioritized over cost-effective preventive interventions. This leads to poor health outcomes and inappropriate care—patients have long waiting periods for care, resulting in worsened health conditions—with unnecessary pain and suffering for people with disabilities, Glassman said. He asked, "How can the participants of this workshop prevent having this same discussion a decade from now?" Glassman suggested the oral health community has an opportunity to fundamentally rethink oral health so prevention, promotion, and care take place in the community while dental offices can serve as the foundation and center of the delivery system. This would bring oral health promotion and disease prevention to those living in underserved communities. Most people could be kept healthy in community locations if the best evidence-based prevention is used, including early intervention and behavior change as supported by science, he said. Providing preventive services in the community could reserve the dental office for complex treatments that could only be performed in that environment.

To get there, Glassman discussed the need for advances in measurement and payment systems, prevention and behavior science, and delivery systems. For measurement and payment systems, he believes it is critical to start focusing on the idea of measuring and providing incentives, and for the health care systems, particularly the oral health care system, on producing population health. There is now a huge opportunity brought about by advances in prevention and behavior support science. Preventive measures include fluoride varnish and silver diamine fluoride, dental sealants and interim therapeutic sequestration. The beauty of these prevention measures is that all these things can be highly effective in controlling dental disease and can be done by someone like a dental hygienist. "You don't need a dentist, you don't need a dental drill, you don't need a dental office," he said. Additionally, Glassman brought up a mistaken belief that information is lacking in telling people to brush their teeth and eat better. The issue is changing behavior, he said, that is the challenge. To achieve behavior change, he suggested having messages delivered by trusted community members, people with similar life circumstances, and those who can provide peer support—that is how to affect behavior change.

Delivery systems are also important, said Glassman. For example, the virtual dental home brings care into communities (Pacific Center for Special Care, 2014). Glassman showed how the model works using an example of a young man, Dennis, with intellectual and developmental disabilities. Dennis was not particularly verbal, although he could speak, but he got nervous in an office, so it became a habit to just use general anesthesia. "That's the way things were done for him," Glassman said. Although when the virtual dental home was used, he was very cooperative receiving oral health preventive care from a dental hygienist in his own living room.

These measures, Glassman stated, are aimed at shortening the inhumane long lines people with disabilities are in to get the dental care they need. Changing the focus could improve the health of communities and people in general. To achieve this, he said it is important to start measuring and providing incentives for outcomes that are population based, not just for clinic attenders. This would foster delivery systems that reach people who do not typically come into dental offices or clinics, he said. Finally, Glassman noted that there is a need to begin to integrate oral health systems to include medical, educational, and social service systems. Each system needs to follow, understand, and use the best evidence-based approaches in procedures and behavior change support. What Glassman envisions are community-engaged oral health systems in which the dental office is not the center of the delivery system, as it currently is. Barriers he sees to achieving this vision include awareness, policies, and moving oral health care providers out of their silos, out of offices and clinics, and into the community where they can integrate with others outside the health system. This would provide an opportunity to change the value equation for oral health, particularly for people with disabilities.

Learning from and with Other Professions to Increase Oral Health Promotion and Disease Prevention

To further address the topic of oral health promotion and disease prevention, a panel of experts from different health professions was invited to speak about their experiences working in this space. Each presenter shared their unique experience as well as interprofessional perspectives on the topic.

Registered Dental Hygienist

Karen Hall is a registered dental hygienist working as an oral health integration manager at Capitol Dental Care in Oregon. She talked about her experiences in two small critical access care hospitals, providing assessments, oral health education, preventive services, and help with post-discharge navigation for patients to receive immediate dental care. In addition to those roles, Hall also helps with dental pain management for patients coming to the emergency room. One observation she shared was that patients who are treated by a team of experts and specialists are likely to receive a more holistic approach to their disease management, health, and recovery. Furthermore, from her interprofessional education experiences, Hall has seen the value of learning from others in the hospital setting.

Hall then described a hospitalized patient with a chronic infection; the medical team was having difficulty locating the source of the infection. A note in the chart said the patient had dental decay and neglect, but it had not been further evaluated. Following several days of hospitalization and not finding the source of the infection, the patient was referred to Hall for an assessment. Hall performed an extensive assessment, including dental X-rays using portable equipment, and discovered that the patient suffered from severe chronic periodontal disease, with three dental abscesses, and teeth that were broken down because of decay. After this assessment, the medical provider was able to prescribe medication appropriate for oral infections, and Hall discussed with the nursing staff the specific oral care needs of the patient to modify the daily care in the hospital. She also talked to the dietitian about the patient's nutritional needs, given the patient's inability to chew solid foods.

Looking beyond the hospital stay, Hall was able to organize a dental appointment for the patient immediately upon discharge. Hall underscored the interprofessional value of dental hygienists in a hospital setting for helping the entire medical team understand the linkages between oral health and patient care that, in the example she shared, led to an earlier discharge from the hospital. But most importantly, Hall emphasized how a culture shift in the hospital had taken place; not only is the medical team working together to help get the patient healthier and out of the hospital, but now the team has also embraced the dental provider as an important member of that team.

Pediatric Nurse Practitioner

The next speaker was Donna M. Hallas, a pediatric nurse practitioner who came to New York University Myers College of Nursing in 2007. When she started at the institution, Hallas was asked to determine how to work interprofessionally with NYU's College of Dentistry, so she met with a pediatric dentist and dental hygienist, and they started working together. As a starting point, their small team performed a literature search to investigate whether there was a need for oral health prevention in newborn care. This turned out to be the case, and they started a study at Bellevue Hospital, in which mothers of children deemed high risk received oral health promotion education. After 6 and 12 months, the children whose mothers received the education showed no sign of dental decay.

Hallas continues to work with the College of Dentistry and has recently focused on individual children and adolescents with disabilities. One advantage of dentists and nurse practitioners working together in this space is that there is no competition for payment. Before embarking on a new project though, Hallas and her team asked, "What are our individual strengths? How can we help each other?" In answering the questions, they realized the 3rd-year nursing students would be able to do comprehensive history taking and teach dental students how to do that, while the dental students could teach the nursing students how to manage and help patients during the dental procedures. Hallas called this a win-win situation.

Physician Assistant

The third speaker, Cynthia Lord, is a physician assistant at the Lake County Free Clinic in Ohio. She shared her perspective as an educator and as someone having worked in an interprofessional oral health space for many years. Lord explained that today most health profession educational programs have an accreditation requirement for interprofessional education. The Interprofessional Education Collaborative (IPEC) was formed in 2009 by six national education associations. IPEC released the first *Core*

Competencies for Interprofessional Collaborative Practice in 2011 (IPEC, 2023). These competencies have provided a framework to help prepare future health professionals for enhanced team-based care for patients and improved population health outcomes. Lord and her team aim to provide health profession students with real-life interprofessional experiences using the four IPEC competency areas of value and ethics, roles and responsibility, communication, and teamwork.

One example Lord described took place when she was at Case Western Reserve, where she worked with an interprofessional team of medical providers as an advisor and preceptor of a student-managed health clinic. In this clinic, student teams of social workers, physician assistants, medical nursing, and dental students see patients using a shared-visit model. At the end of each clinic, the students evaluate their teamwork and provide feedback to one another using a case-developed tool based on direct observation of team interaction. Another example is the Case Western Reserve's collaborative practice course, which is required for all 1st-year medical, dental, physician assistant, social work, and speech-language pathology students, as well as 4th-year nursing students. The students spend 2 hours each week during two semesters working in small teams with students from different professions. Lord noted that half of the time is spent learning about teamwork, problem solving, conflict management, providing and receiving feedback, and the relevance to their future careers. These skills are then applied in the other half of the time while working in the community on a project with a local agency. At the end of the project, each team presents their project to the leadership from the community agency as part of the collaborative practice showcase. Lord said that these examples demonstrate how deep learning from and with other health professions can happen.

Registered Dietitian Nutritionist

Teresa A. Marshall is a professor of preventive and community dentistry at the University of Iowa and works as a dietitian. Marshall explained how the diet-to-oral health interface is bidirectional. She said that a poor diet increases the risk of oral disease, which leads to tooth and soft-tissue loss, making it harder to bite, chew, and swallow whole grains and fruit and vegetables, which make up a healthy diet.

Marshall added that poor oral health is associated with nutrient-poor diets, which exacerbates the risk of systemic disease. Rather than just focusing on dietary modification to reduce sugars in a patient with existing caries, it would be far more cost-effective to identify dietary risk factors in patients with a healthy mouth as a way of preventing disease.

Marshall also discussed how dietitians are involved with modifying textures, food compositions, and meal patterns for patients with limited oral motor skills associated with some disabilities. For individuals with inborn errors of metabolism, or those using medications with oral side effects, such as decreased saliva, extensive dietary modifications may be necessary to ensure adequate nutrient intake and to reduce the risk of caries.

Dietitians and oral health care professionals cannot work alone to prevent oral disease, said Marshall. Bringing the larger health community into a conversation can help spread the message that diet-related risk factors are the same for oral and systemic diseases, which can both be addressed as a team. Ideally, such a health care team would be composed of dentists, hygienists, dietitians, physicians, social workers, psychologists, community workers, and others to send a common dietary message to people, she said. This requires interdisciplinary training so every team member understands dental disease and how each can help facilitate prevention. Marshall finished her remarks by explaining that at the societal level, there is a need to create policies addressing the social determinants of health, such that healthy diets become the preferred choice and are available to all.

Health Psychologist

Daniel W. McNeil is the chair of the Department of Community Dentistry and Behavioral Science at the University of Florida. McNeil works as a health psychologist, and in his department, public health dentists, dental hygienists, and psychologists all work together. He explained that this type of collaboration results in a synergy that can be used for the goals of this workshop. He further commented that behavior is often discussed in terms of patients and prevention; however, other types of behavior are also crucially important, such as the behavior of providers, policy makers, and payers. This is how clinical health psychology can play a part in working together with other professions to change behavior at various levels, he said.

McNeil then asked the workshop participants to think about what all the speakers talked about, which was *behavior*, mainly as it relates to patients and prevention, although the behavior of providers and others is arguably even more important. For example, Paul Glassman talked about the response of dental providers to having individuals with disabilities come to their offices; Helen Lee talked about what people are doing in their daily lives. The behavior of providers and their personnel who support them, McNeil believes, is crucially important, and this is how clinical health psychology can be a part of the team working with other professions to change behavior at various levels. The behavior of policy makers and payers is another group that can have profound implications for the integration of care. In 2022, McNeil and others published a consensus statement on the role of behavioral and social sciences in oral health (McNeil et al., 2022). In it, the authors underscored the importance of embracing collaborations to achieve the goals set for interprofessional work in order to change the paradigm in dentistry.

DIALOGUE WITH THE INTERPROFESSIONAL PANELISTS

During a discussion with the audience that followed, an online participant asked about strategies to ensure that core competencies are centered around the patient and family experience: "How do you ensure this work meets the standard of 'nothing about us, without us' as wished for by people with disabilities?" Garcia answered that each academic unit has different standards to meet from various accreditors, and as dental educators, it has been helpful that there is an expectation to have interprofessional education that constitutes real engagement of students early in the curriculum. From the first day of becoming a dental student and throughout the curriculum, students meet and engage with other health professions. It is not a didactic exercise but one that takes interprofessional teams of students into the community for hands-on experiences, she said. To make that happen, Garcia emphasized the importance of making every encounter meaningful and practical, so students value the experience and develop interprofessional skills to take with them as they go into their various health professions.

Lee commented that in PROTECT, which is a community-informed clinical trial to change the behaviors of the surgical population as mentioned above, the study team realized that to help families change their behaviors that the team needed to understand what was going on in households of these families. The protocol included extensive formative assessments. Several interviews were conducted with community health workers, who were the interventionists for the trial, and had experience working in the West and South Side of Chicago, serving the families that were representative of the trial's target population. Lee and her team also interviewed families who were coming into the hospital for their child's care, and they interviewed pediatric dentists rooted in the communities. Then they ran the protocol, including everything from recruitment to flyers to retain participants. Through the community engagement advisory board they received feedback and hired research assistants who were undergraduates from the same neighborhoods.

Lord described work at her institution where students obtain experience not in a lecture or classroom but by practicing in the community as part of a team. The students are taught the IPEC competencies and use those in the field. Communication is important for this, as well as values and ethics. That is how, from the very beginning, students work with clients in the community and learn the importance of respect for patient and colleagues so when they become professionals this is already embedded within them. It is not something they learned about but instead something they grew up with and internalized.

Hall commented that working in a dental care organization that employs dental hygienists and community workers, it is obvious to her who has had interprofessional training. Those who are taught and have experienced positive collaborations across professions are more likely to facilitate those relationships in settings such as hospitals or other medical settings where the health professions collocate with dental team members. In her experience, people who have received the training are generally more eager to make those interprofessional relationships work.

Glassman added his thoughts on how to better integrate the voices of the community. A system of educating students with some kind of experience and then hoping they use it when they graduate often does not translate into real-world changes in the way dentistry is most often practiced. He said there is another way to think about it, both within and outside of educational institutions. Community structures, he reiterated, need to be integrated with other kinds of systems and pay attention to the voice of the community, develop systems that work, and then expose students to those. This is from an opposite starting point, with an emphasis on building community delivery systems. He thinks that dental education institutions have a role in exposing students to community-level health systems, which is the opposite approach from thinking about the starting point being educating students differently. Glassman believes in starting by changing the delivery systems and then letting students see what that looks like.

An audience member from Pacific Dental Services asked Glassman whether he envisioned patients themselves providing the dental prevention measures as discussed, such as sealants and fluoride varnish. Glassman responded by saying this is something that could happen, and anything that can be done to push forward preventive measures, in terms of procedures and behavior change and daily mouth care, is the right direction. Products in use now likely will not be deregulated, but in California there is a law stating that anybody can apply fluoride varnish; it does not have to be a dental professional. The caveat is that this person has to be in some program, trained, and monitored by a dentist. However, this is not the case in many states.

Placing emphasis on programs where support can be provided to people for incorporating effective innovations that become daily routines is the way to go, according to Glassman. Such innovations could bring oral health care into elementary schools. Glassman and his colleagues performed a 6-year demonstration of the idea of a virtual dental home with hygienists in elementary schools. Findings from the project showed that by using this model, low-income children with high disease rates could be kept healthy at school without needing to go to a dental office. The dentist was involved through a virtual review of records taken by the hygienist. This model is effective, said Glassman, but there is currently a lack of awareness, policy, and implementation to support bringing this and similar disease prevention models for oral health into practice.

Michael, who identifies as a person with disabilities from the Arc of Philadelphia, asked,

> If the panelists were able to change the system, how would they go about getting more funding for the whole dental system so that everybody can get health care? What should be asked from the government to get more federal funding for the whole dental community?

Garcia responded that this question gets to the heart of the matter—advocating for funding. The ideas are there, she said, but systems would need to be developed, along with funding to support the system. When thinking about funding, Garcia felt it was important to think about all the interested groups and the community, noting that it would be helpful to see concerted efforts from the federal government focusing specifically on this. There is also a great opportunity to engage local agencies and nonprofit organizations. Garcia suggested there is a need to look broadly and try to engage more individuals to provide more funding opportunities. Whether these are local, state level, or from the dental industry, funding is what can help move many of the ideas proposed at this workshop.

Lord echoed Garcia's call for funding but answered Michael's question by asking people in the United States to value their mouth as much as their overall health. "The people in this country need to stand up and tell Washington that this is important to them," she said, "because they [policy makers] think we all have an ulterior motive, that we all want more money, we want more power, whatever it might be."

McNeil also commented on the funding aspect saying this may be another case for interprofessional activity:

> Not only must dentists and dental hygienists speak up, but it is also important for consumers, patients, public advocacy groups, and other professional groups to say oral health is important and related to general health.

That, McNeil believes, would be a more persuasive message and goes back to the behavior of policy makers—how can their behavior in policy making be influenced?

Glassman reflected on the discussion before commenting that there is not really a need for more money. The issue is how the money is spent. In oral health, too much is spent on general anesthesia and on late-stage repair, said Glassman, so the problem is not spending the finances correctly.

Glassman called it a bucket problem, where if money is saved in hospitalization, it does not go back to the dental providers. Rethinking dental care delivery systems and getting to people earlier in the disease process would allow for the wiser use of funds and could produce better health for the population at lower costs.

3

Understanding the Value Proposition in Oral Health

BOX 3-1
Key Points Made by Individual Speakers[*]

- A value proposition solves pain or enhances gains for all the vested interest groups. (Berman)
- The practice of not accepting people with disabilities into dental practices and referring them to the hospital for anesthesia, which is currently often done, is the easier way, but it is inhumane and inappropriate. (Kemp)
- The value proposition for providers is the importance of improved health through prevention. Oral health is an example that crosses essentially all body systems. (Deutchman)
- Payers have a role to play in making a meaningful contribution to the management of oral health and medical health, as well as overall integration—a key part of a payer's value proposition. (Tillman)
- Value in value-based care refers to what an individual values most. From there, it is possible to design care coordination so it achieves the target of improved outcomes. (Chalmers)
- Preventive care is often not covered by insurance or Medicaid programs. (Wolff)
- A sensory-adapted dental environment for children with autism spectrum disorders significantly improved physiological distress and behavioral distress, while not decreasing the quality of care. (Stein Duker)
- A 2023 caries risk assessment found that 72 percent of the patients were at high risk for dental caries and the cost of sending a patient to the operating room for dental care could be avoided if they could receive preventive care more than a couple of times a year. (White)

[*]This list is the rapporteurs' summary of points made by the individual speakers identified, and the statements have not been endorsed or verified by the National Academies of Sciences, Engineering, and Medicine. They are not intended to reflect a consensus among workshop participants.

The next workshop session aimed at providing attendees and speakers with a better understanding of what a value proposition in oral health could look like. Robert Weyant, associate dean of Dental Public Health and Community Outreach at the University of Pittsburgh, chaired the session. In his remarks, he framed the upcoming presentation and discussion saying, "We will embark on a journey to examine the profound impact of oral health on diverse vested interest groups beyond the traditional lens of dental care." He asked attendees to keep in mind the value of prevention, a core part of patient care and system design. The value of disease prevention can lead to lower costs, improved health and well-being, program sustainability, and enhanced quality of life, he said.

VALUE PROPOSITION FOR ORAL HEALTH

Richard Berman, associate vice president for strategic initiatives for innovation and research at the University of South Florida, described a value proposition as it relates to oral health. "It's that thing that is so obviously important ... why isn't it happening?" he asked. He went on to answer his question with "[It is] because people don't value it the same way you value it and the same way you see it so obviously." Berman emphasized that different people value oral health differently. For a value proposition in oral health, one would be looking for a sustainable solution that will make an improvement. It is important to determine who the customer is. For example, he said, if someone were to build a startup selling a new product, it would be important to realize who the customer is. If the customer does not see value in the new product being offered, it will not sell, and the startup would not be sustainable. Therefore, the value proposition should look for a sustainable solution that improves the oral health of the population.

Berman discussed a business model with various segments, which is used by the National Science Foundation and many venture capital groups to decide what new projects or programs to fund. This business model is also being taught in universities. To understand the value proposition, it is important to realize that it caters to the requirements of a specific customer segment, and therefore based on those segments' differentiated needs and or behaviors. Rather than creating an intricate business plan, leaders often summarize their hypotheses in a framework called a business model canvas. Essentially, this is a diagram of how a company will create value for itself and its customers (Figure 3-1).

In health care, there are three main vested interest groups or segments, he said. The first are the patients, the clients, or the community. This goes back to the earlier-mentioned statement of "you cannot do something for us, without us." For these groups, it will be important to ask what people

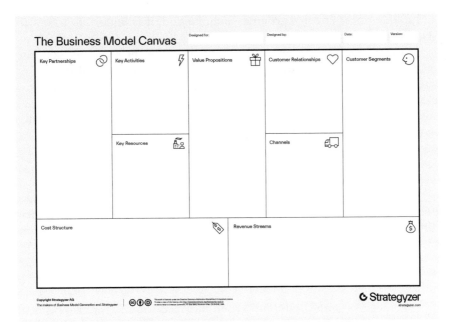

FIGURE 3-1 The business model canvas.
SOURCE: Berman presentation, February 15, 2024. Illustration created by Strategyzer AG (strategyzer.com). This work is licensed under the Creative Commons Attribution-ShareAlike 3.0 Unported License. To view a copy of this license, visit http://creativecommons.org/licenses/by-sa/3.0/.

with physical or cognitive disabilities or conditions need. Aspects to think about in this respect are payments, access to a place, relief from fear or anxiety, and whether there is access in the evening or only during the day. There is a need to understand who the patient or end user or community is and consider language, money, culture, and other factors, he said. To determine the answers to these questions, Berman stated that it is essential to go to patients and clients and ask open-ended questions. The most important part of the value proposition is to understand from those who have a vested interest in the issue what their problem is that the value proposition aims to resolve or improve.

Berman noted that the second vested interest group in health care consists of providers and educators. For this group, it is important to understand what their barrier or problem is and what their gain is. Again, it is critical to ask this group what is important to them to ensure that the proposed solution meets their issue. Finally, the third group is the payers, which can be insurers, Medicare, Medicaid or other government programs, and foundations. For this group as well, he said, it is important to understand their pains and gains.

Berman finalized his explanation of the value proposition, confirming that one would be looking for a value proposition that solves pain or enhances gains for all the interested parties (Figure 3-2). When there is a clear understanding of customer satisfaction for a product or service, a solution can be devised that matches the value proposition, which results in the building of a sustainable model.

Perspectives from Groups with a Vested Interest

To better understand the oral health value proposition, four speakers presented their views on the pains and gains from the perspectives of their different groups: (1) persons with disabilities, (2) providers and educators, (3) payers, and (4) policy makers.

Persons with Disabilities

The persons with disabilities group member, John Kemp, is president and chief executive officer of the Lakeshore Foundation and is part of the people with disabilities community. He discussed projects on accessible oral health in response to the question: What better ways are there to serve people with disabilities for improving oral health, and thus, overall health?

Kemp said that asking for equity in health care distribution is important. Disability has now been recognized as a health disparity by the U.S. Department of Health and Human Services (NIH, 2023). To improve this disparity, it is essential to look for respect and inclusion in all aspects of care, he said. Inclusion requires a different way of serving people, and the minimum should be access and equality overall. In the community, there

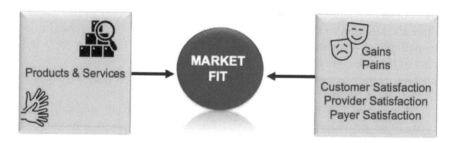

FIGURE 3-2 The value proposition should solve pains and enhance gains for each vested interest group.
SOURCE: Berman presentation, February 15, 2024.

is the issue of accessibility of the dental office. Further, he emphasized the need for culturally competent people to serve the needs of people with disabilities, which requires education and training. The practice of not accepting people with disabilities into dental practices and referring them to the hospital for anesthesia, which is currently often done, is the easier way, Kemp said, but it is inhumane and inappropriate.

Another accessibility issue is that many dental offices use portals to access information. In order for this to work, the patient has to be able to access the portal, and have Internet service, phones, and other tools, which can be a barrier in terms of costs or usability. Additional barriers, Kemp said, include the way providers communicate with patients and clients. This should be done in an accessible format, but this is not always the case. For example, when video is used as an instructional tool, it would be important to also have it captioned so it is accessible, and people can make choices on how they receive the information.

There is also the issue of culture. While 17 percent of the population with disabilities are born with the disability, the majority—83 percent—acquire the disability through injury, illness, accidents, or other events. To these people, the disability and its barriers are new, as they are to their family and caregivers. Therefore, it can be challenging for this group to negotiate their needs and navigate the system, Kemp said. He noted that people with disabilities now demand the respect that is essential for them to ask for equality and equity; a heightened acceptance of human differences is essential for this.

Finally, Kemp noted some barriers that exist for people with disabilities receiving oral health preventive care. For instance, to get to a dental office, barriers may exist in terms of transportation, accessibility of the dental office, and acceptance by dental providers. People might make it to a dental office and get turned down after having spent money and time to get there. Another barrier is communication, with some in health care talking condescendingly to people with disabilities. For people with disabilities, these types of accessibility barriers provide a silent message that they are not being welcomed, said Kemp. In closing, Kemp emphasized that "what we're really looking for is respect and inclusion in all aspects." He added that persons with disabilities are not asking for more than their fair share, just equity in the health care distribution that, in this case, would make the dental office fully accessible and free of barriers for all people.

Providers and Educators (Interprofessional)

As a physician with a rural practice background, Mark Deutchman, the associate dean for rural health at the University of Colorado, presented virtually about what he sees as the value proposition for health care providers and educators, with particular focus on interdisciplinary practice and education, and on persons with disabilities.

Deutchman first discussed the value proposition for providers. For them, he said, there is the importance of improved health through prevention. Providers are looking for ways within the scope of their care and abilities to prevent disease and disability. Oral health is an example of a tool that crosses essentially all body systems. Deutchman underscored the importance of the link between oral health and overall health and that much of oral disease is preventable via personal behaviors. When this is understood, he said, it becomes intuitive that mechanisms to promote oral health and prevent dental and related diseases should be adopted. Examples include looking for ways to connect virtually for counseling patients about what they can do for themselves and performing interventions available within the practice environment and scope of care. Although Deutchman is not a dentist, he can look in the mouth and identify gum disease. He can also teach students to look for spots that might identify dental caries. Furthermore, he can apply fluoride varnish, and soon he may be able to apply silver diamine fluoride; train students, residents, and fellows; and collaborate with other health and nonhealth professionals so everyone is able to perform these tasks.

For health care providers, said Deutchman, something like fluoride varnish for kids is an attractive intervention because it works and because it is preventive. It is also important for health care providers to realize that when treating people with disabilities and chronic illness, prescribed medications can adversely affect oral health.

Deutchman then shifted to say that health care providers already do things such as motivational interviewing with people regarding tobacco, seat belts, helmets, and reproductive health, and these same skills are transferable to talk about oral health. The skillset is there, he asserts. Once the knowledge and desire to include prevention and health promotion messages to people and populations is in place, change can happen; however, Deutchman acknowledged that there are barriers. Change does not happen without administrative buy-in, and all providers have time constraints, he said. This means that administrators who do the hiring and determine schedules must value the messaging as well.

For educators, the value proposition constitutes a curriculum opportunity for interprofessional education although a major barrier to making this happen is the already overflowing curriculum. As a result, it becomes hard for educators to introduce a new module, subject, or class, he noted. However, since oral health crosses various subjects and disciplines (e.g., anatomy, infectious disease, nutrition, aging, special needs, disabilities, and metabolism), the topic could be introduced by, for example, asking a simple question like, "What is *Streptococcus mutans*?" This is how students could start to learn about oral health while also providing interprofessional, experiential learning opportunities. If students learn with and from colleagues from other professions while they are in training, concluded Deutchman, there is a better chance they will practice collaboratively and use the interpersonal skills they acquired during training after graduation.

Payers

Randi Tillman, executive dental director, Health Care Services Corporation (HCSC) attended virtually and discussed the value proposition for insurers. She noted at the start of her talk that experience has taught her that value is in the "eyes of the beholder," and depends heavily on the individual's perspective. As someone who works in insurance, Tillman shared her views from that lens saying, "Yes, of course we are interested in the [return on investment], but we are also interested in our public image and in gaining a competitive advantage." For insurers, it is important to manage health care costs—both medical and dental—for their customers, Tillman said. Their customers are employer groups, but insurers are also committed to improving overall health and are aware that they are selling very personal products.

As an organization, Tillman said, it strives to be an industry leader in oral health and medical dental integration, which means the company wants to learn how to do things better. Many patients have both medical and dental coverage with HCSC, allowing for integrated care. As an insurer, HCSC can provide additional dental benefits, which can help manage both medical diagnosis and the oral environment. This does not typically result in any extra effort or cost for the patient, said Tillman. HCSC tries to incentivize the use of these additional benefits by their clients. For instance, HCSC staff can remind patients with diabetes and cardiovascular disease to maintain their oral health by sending postcards and providing phone call reminders. The same goes for dental patients who the company knows have chronic medical conditions; they too can receive company reminders.

Tillman explained that when employers are looking to purchase medical and dental insurance, the most significant cost is on the medical side. Therefore, she said that an argument can be made that if good oral health is maintained, the costs on the medical side can be reduced. This has been backed by some research, Tillman noted, that has shown that patients with chronic medical conditions who receive regular preventive dental care experience better medical outcomes. However, she also noted that exacerbation of chronic illness is multifactorial, which means that poor dental care can be a contributor, but it is often not the sole contributing factor. Tillman concluded by saying that payers have a role to play in making a meaningful contribution to the management of oral health and medical health, as well as overall integration—a key part of a payer's value proposition.

After finishing her remarks, a question was posed whether teledentistry could be used for preventive dental checks for bridging the gap in oral health care use in children. Robert Weyant noted that there is variability in teledentistry policy and the ability to use it between states, which poses a barrier. John Kemp added how essential it is that any technology also be accessible to parents who are deaf or need someone to type for them. Whichever way it is delivered, he noted, the technology would have to be accessible to all. Michael Helgeson said that telehealth can be great for many different groups of people. For dental care, a large amount of work can be done where the person lives, where they go to school, or where they work. This can solve lots of problems, and advice can be provided to patients. Providing care in the community lifts many of the barriers discussed for people with disabilities in getting to dental offices although also using telehealth before an office visit can save money and time and create better patient experiences, he said.

Policy Makers

Natalia I. Chalmers is the chief dental officer at the Office of the Administrator at the Centers for Medicare and Medicaid Services (CMS). As a pediatric dentist and oral health policy expert, Chalmers guides CMS in advancing oral health in Medicaid, the Children's Health Insurance Program (CHIP), Marketplace, and Medicare. In her talk, she highlighted the effect of the programs at CMS that provide health coverage for close to 160 million people in the United States, of which 88.4 million are insured through Medicaid and CHIP (CMS, n.d.a). CMS is committed to serving the public as a trusted partner and steward, said Chalmers. CMS is dedicated to advancing health equity, expanding coverage, and improving health outcomes for all people including persons with disabilities. More specifically, Chalmers regards CMS as a steward of value-based payment models while also managing a variety of crosscutting initiatives that are multiyear endeavors. One of these initiatives was launched in the past year and focuses on oral health. The initiative considers every opportunity to expand access to oral health coverage using existing authorities and health plan flexibilities.

When people do not have access to a dental care delivery system, they will end up in the broader health care system for emergency care (Figure 3-3). The dental care delivery system depicted on the left of the figure, shows that many people in the United States regularly visit their dentist, often on a 6-month schedule, said Chalmers, thereby limiting or avoiding the need for emergency dental care. However, further to the right

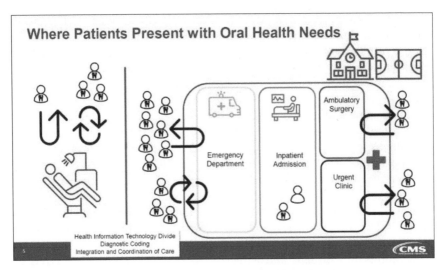

FIGURE 3-3 Where patients present with oral health needs.
SOURCE: Chalmers presentation, February 16, 2024. Image created by Chalmers.

are a variety of scenarios where emergency care is used, such as when a child with a painful tooth abscess is brought to the emergency room for care. Some people are repeat users of emergency care—shown as circular arrows—while others who are admitted for a variety of nondental conditions also suffer from poor oral health that can negatively affect their overall health outcome. Chalmers then pointed to the right side of the figure saying ambulatory surgical clinics and urgent care clinics provide additional points of entry into the health system and could be opportunities for preventing oral disease and promoting oral health. These messages can also be spread through community organizations such as schools and recreational facilities.

Further underscoring the financial burden of treating people with dental disease versus preventing it, Chalmers asked, "Is this the best use of resources given the high cost of care in the emergency departments and the low cost of oral disease prevention?" She asked the audience to realize the effect of poor oral health on patients who are admitted for other surgeries; financial burden is not only about the dental problem driving people to hospital emergency care, but it is also that poor dental health can affect surgical outcomes.

Chalmers noted that coverage is only the first step; getting to and finding providers that can address the needs of people is more complicated. Another barrier is the health information technology divide. It can be hard for small-scale dental practices to overcome that challenge and connect to a large health care system or an electronic health record. Therefore, providers in those settings must rely on the medical information that the patient recalls. This might not be very accurate, and patients may not realize the link between certain conditions and oral health. For instance, the use of some antidepressants can result in xerostomia (dry mouth), which affects oral health.

Diagnostic coding was mentioned earlier as a barrier, and there is no standard of practice. Chalmers said it is important that all health care providers speak the same language to truly understand each other. These factors all affect the coordination of care, she said.

Referencing data from the Health Policy Institute, Chalmers showed progress made for children. However, the data show a gap between children who live below the federal poverty guidelines and those who do not in terms of how often they visit the dentist. This gap is closing, but the difference is still approximately 20 percent, and the gap is even bigger for older adults (Yarbrough and Vujicic, 2019). Chalmers then referred to data from 2018 showing that some people only see a dentist (8.6 percent), some only see a physician (34.4 percent), some see both (37.1 percent), and some see neither (19.8 percent) (Manski et al., 2021). If the dentist is the only access to care, there is a huge opportunity to do more medically, such as screening for blood pressure or diabetes, she said. Data show that coverage matters for these issues, but even when it is limited or not there, people end up needing dental care (Manski et al., 2022).

Chalmers followed up her comments with National Health Expenditure data on dental health costs showing such costs represent 4 percent of the total expenditures, or $165 billion (CMS, 2023). On average, the out-of-pocket spending is approximately 40 percent, while the rest of health care is around 9 percent. For Medicare beneficiaries in the community, this percentage is even higher. Chalmers said that this is one of the biggest barriers to accessing dental care.

Chalmers then discussed definitions for value-based care and associated terminology as defined by the CMS Center for Innovation (CMS, n.d.b). She noted that it is important to define what is meant by accountable care—a person-centered care team takes responsibility for improving the quality of care, care coordination, and health outcomes for a defined group of individuals, to reduce care fragmentation and avoid unnecessary costs for individuals and the health system. Care coordination is the organization of an individual's care across multiple health care providers. Integrated care can be defined as an approach to coordinate health care services to better address an individual's physical, mental, behavioral, and social needs, while person-centered care consists of integrated health care services delivered in a setting and manner that is responsive to individuals and their goals, values, and preferences in a system that supports good provider–patient communication and empowers individuals receiving care and providers to make effective care plans together.

Chalmers defined value-based care as designing care so it focuses on quality, provider performance, and the patient experience. Therefore, the *value* in value-based care refers to what an individual values most. From there, it is possible to design care coordination so it achieves the target of improved outcomes, she said.

The CMS Innovation Center develops and implements payment and service delivery models (pilot programs) and conducts congressionally mandated demonstrations to support health care transformation and increase access to high-quality care, said Chalmers.

Chalmers noted that at the heart of value-based care is reliable measurement. Additionally, it is essential to understand that barriers to care and the health goals of individuals can only be uncovered by talking to the individuals themselves. She argued that health goals cannot be assumed and can only be uncovered by listening, particularly to caregivers and persons with disabilities who are the recipients of the care.

An online audience member asked Chalmers to share her thoughts about mid-level dental providers that could be implemented in dentistry in various settings. Chalmers said that such decisions are made at the state level. State governments decide who is eligible to practice in their states. Another virtual participant asked how the oral health field could become accessible to disabled practitioners. Chalmers noted that it is important to understand how disability is defined. For instance, providers, both dental and nondental, struggle with mental health challenges and some may have some level of disability. Helgeson added that dental practitioners can limit their practice in different ways to account for their various kinds of disabilities.

DEMONSTRATING THE VALUE PROPOSITION
FOR PERSONS WITH DISABILITIES

Mark Wolff, dean of Penn Dental Medicine, moderated the session exploring an oral health value proposition for persons with disabilities. He opened by describing the program at Penn Dental Medicine in which students spend 20 percent of their time in the community doing dentistry in an interprofessional medical setting, and 10 percent of their time at Penn Dental Medicine's Center for Persons with Disabilities. The goal of the program is to learn from and with other professions while becoming comfortable working with people who have a variety of different disabilities. A goal of the program is for students to learn how to deliver the best care and communicate with caregivers and patients so 90 to 95 percent of individuals coming to the center can be treated without sedation or general anesthesia. The personalized care suite sees 8,000 patients per year in that facility, Wolff said, and Penn Dental Medicine trains 200 dentists a year and additionally provides continuing education to tens of thousands. The school has immersion projects with individuals who can come to the school and learn how to deliver this care after taking continuing education.

For treatment, Wolff argued it is very important to discuss equity and equality in treatment. Overall, he said, real change is needed, and it should not be the goal to make a rotten system a bit less rotten. CareQuest recently published outcomes associated with oral health showing that oral health affects activities of daily living, how people eat, concentrate, sleep, and learn (Heaton et al., 2024). When it comes to value-based care, Wolff noted it is also essential to discuss productivity hours lost due to unexpected emergency dental visits and oral pain. The report estimated 13 million adults lost 187 million productivity hours annually. Further, 5.7 million parents and caregivers lost 243 million productivity hours caused by unexpected emergencies. Therefore, Wolff said, it is important to consider the real costs of poor oral health.

Wolff then asked, "Where are people with disabilities going to find care?" He said preventive care is often not covered by insurance or Medicaid programs. Penn Dental Medicine writes off approximately $3 million annually in preventive and supplemental visits that are not covered. There are other financial costs as well, such as emergency room visits and care in operating rooms, but also the cost to society when opioids are prescribed for mouth pain that lead to addiction. Wolff emphasized that including these sorts of costs should be considered when talking about value-based care. The cost is not the payment of $18 per patient for providing fluoride varnish to prevent decay, he argued, and value-based care should take the real savings seen throughout the system and distribute them back to caregivers and the care system to reduce overall cost. However, Wolff acknowledges that this will be very challenging to do.

Creating Sensory-Adapted Dental Environments for Children with Autism Spectrum Disorders

The first session speaker was Leah Stein Duker, assistant professor at the University of Southern California Chan Division of Occupational Science and Occupational Therapy. Presenting virtually, Stein Duker shared her work in creating sensory-adapted dental environments for children with autism spectrum disorders (ASD) that she used as a case example for an oral health value proposition. She described the pain points for children with ASD that can lead to overreactions to stimulation and can be exhibited as fight-or-flight reactions. The difficulties may be induced by auditory stimuli (caused by dental equipment or a crowded office), tactile stimuli (such as feeling on face and inside of the mouth by a dentist's gloved hand and their equipment), olfactory stimuli (resulting from the taste and smell of the prophylactic paste, fluoride varnish, dentist gloves, and even the perfume of the provider), vestibular movement stimuli (from the feeling of reclining back in a chair), and visual stimuli (caused by bright lights in the clinic and the overall visually distracting environment). Stein Duker shared that these differences in sensory processing stimuli are so common in the ASD population that it was added to the DSM five diagnostic criteria for the condition.

To address the sensory overstimulation, Stein Duker developed an intervention with a multidisciplinary team targeting those sensory experiences during a preventive dental care visit. The resulting sensory-adapted dental environment tackled the various stimuli. To develop this intervention, a team, including people with backgrounds in occupational therapy, dentistry, and psychology, was assembled. The adapted environment modifies the visual, auditory, and tactile stimuli of the dental office. For instance, the overhead lighting was switched off, darkening curtains were placed over the windows, and the dentists used a headlamp to direct the light into the mouth, not the eyes. In addition to the soothing audio and visuals played in the room, a pediatric X-ray bib was used to provide extra weight, and a wrap gave the child tactile deep pressure sensations to provide a calming effect on the nervous system. To assess its effects, a randomized controlled trial was performed including 220 children with ASD between the ages of 6 and 12 years (Stein Duker et al., 2023). Each child had two visits for dental cleaning, one with and one without the environmental changes. Stein Duker found that the adapted environment resulted in significant improvements in physiological distress and behavioral distress, while it did not decrease the quality of care. Furthermore, she found there were no differences in cost-related variables, and it resulted in high satisfaction for caregivers and children.

Stein Duker recognized that her findings were part of a study but noted that it is feasible to implement these low-cost interventions in the real world as this method is highly scalable. Minimal training is required for its implementation, and the modifications do not require clinic renovations, with only a one-time cost. The method is now included in the American Academy of Pediatric Dentistry's list of best practices for behavioral guidance as a potential technique to use with patients with anxiety or special health care needs (American Academy of Pediatric Dentistry, 2023).

During the audience question-and-answer period, Stein Duker was asked if this would also work for adults. Stein Duker said this has not yet been researched for autistic adults, but it is part of her plans to investigate. It has been pilot-tested with success for adults with intellectual and developmental disabilities. Another audience member inquired about the importance of training and whether staff training would be needed on top of the additional costs to the environmental changes? She replied that the process requires minimal training to implement, is easily portable, does not require renovations to the clinic, and it has only a one-time cost associated with it, which could easily be decreased from the $6,000 that she and her colleagues spent in conducting the study. A final audience question inquired what can be done for patients who are already traumatized from past experiences? Stein Duker responded that each individual is unique and would require tailored adaptations, but a good starting point would be to provide a graphic depiction before treatment of all the steps that will happen so the patient knows what to expect. Wolff then asked Stein Duker if her team had done anything related to home care with the caregivers to assist them in routine home care? Stein Duker said they did not, but plan to do that. Training parents would help for things like low-texture, low-taste toothpaste to reduce sensory issues, she noted, and would require using the shared expertise between occupational therapy and dentistry.

Onsite Mobile Oral Health for People with Disabilities

Betsy Lee White is chief operating officer at Access Dental Care, a mobile special care dentistry practice that serves people with disabilities and older adults in North Carolina. White discussed a 24-year effort that began as a pilot project. Her organization provides comprehensive, mobile dental care to individuals in skilled nursing homes, group homes for those with intellectual and developmental disabilities, Program of All-Inclusive Care for the Elderly (PACE) participants, and community-dwelling individuals that are behaviorally or medically complex. The project operates as a nonprofit organization, and has support from the North Carolina Dental Society and other locally interested groups. Its goal is to take the dental office to the community. To do this, a team made up of a dentist, dental hygienist, and two dental assistants—with support from social workers and a logistics coordinator—goes into the community 5 days a week. Seventy percent of the activities performed in the program are diagnostic and preventive services, 10 percent are oral surgeries and extractions, 12 percent are "drill and fill," and 5 percent of the team's work is related to dental partials, which are removable dental appliances used to replace missing teeth.

White then presented data collected by her and her team in 2023 on caries risk assessment as part of CareQuest Institute's initiative on community oral health transformation. Their results showed that 72 percent of the patients they included were at high risk for dental caries. White emphasized the potential cost savings if the people in this study could receive preventive care more than a couple of times a year. "The reimbursement for that would add up to $652," she noted, which would be significantly lower than the roughly $10,000 she estimated it would cost for sending the same person to the operating room for dental care.

Patients in the community with special health care needs face many barriers. The example she used was a patient with multiple sclerosis who was previously refused at a dental office because they were in a wheelchair. White said her team was able to treat this patient, but the paperwork may take months to go through the system. White underscored the need for a system that allows groups like hers to work with people who have intellectual or developmental disabilities or other special health care needs. "We know how to do this," she said. "We just need a system that allows it."

During the discussion, White received a question about compensation. Her response was that if they were reimbursed for all the services they provide, it would bring in an extra $2 million, which would help them grow. Wolff then asked where the funding for their work came from and whether it was based mostly on charitable donations or grants? White said they started the program with grants, but they work to make sure that their clinical operations are self-sustaining. This is becoming a bigger challenge, she remarked, as the reimbursement rate in North Carolina has gone down. "We are below the reimbursement rate that we [had] in 2008 and that equals 34 cents on the dollar."

VESTED INTEREST GROUP INPUT ON A POTENTIAL VALUE PROPOSITION

Richard Berman introduced the next session saying, "To have an effective program or a new project that is sustainable and meaningful, the needs of the interested groups have to be recognized." This constitutes the value to the groups. To explore an oral health value proposition, Berman described the two-part process through which three randomly assigned breakout groups first met to discuss an oral health value proposition before transitioning to a self-identified interest group in the second half of the allotted time. The three groups were (1) persons with disabilities, (2) educators and providers, and (3) payers and policy makers. Coleaders of the three groups presented discussions from their breakout group conversations on their interest group's pains and gains that would make up an oral health value proposition for their target group.

Persons with Disabilities

The breakout group discussing the pains (Table 3-1) and gains (Table 3-2) for persons with disabilities was led by Teresa A. Marshall and Daniel W. McNeil. From the discussion, McNeil said, it became clear that the pains were related to access and ability to find professional dental care.

TABLE 3-1 Oral Health Value Proposition Pains for Persons with Disabilities

PAIN	RATIONALE
Access or ability to find care	Ability to find adequate care; transportation or office accessibility; hidden copays and/or added costs
Demands on caregivers	Burnout; buy-in and prioritization (e.g., nutrition)
Value of oral health care	Prioritization; understanding importance

SOURCE: Presentation by Marshall and McNeil, February 16, 2024.

TABLE 3-2 Oral Health Value Proposition Gains for Persons with Disabilities

GAIN	RATIONALE
Improved quality of life	Acknowledge impact of oral health on physical/systemic health
Advances in materials and technology	Easier delivery of and access to care; teledentistry
Progress toward inclusion	Improvements in awareness, acceptance, and acknowledgment; change in policies

SOURCE: Presentation by Marshall and McNeil, February 16, 2024.

Adequate care is difficult to find for this group, and there are often long waits to see a provider. Furthermore, access is also limited by hidden copays and difficulty in getting to dental care offices in terms of transportation and accessibility of the dental office and building.

A second pain point for persons with disabilities is the demand it adds to caregivers. Many caregivers are having issues with burnout stemming from the psychological demands of their responsibilities and their overwhelming concern for the health and welfare of their family members or the person with whom they are working. The third mentioned pain point was the view on the value of oral health care, or the prioritization of oral health. Persons with disabilities and their caregivers often have many competing priorities in life, including other health care problems, and there might be limited understanding of the importance of oral health for overall health.

The possible gains for persons with disabilities for oral health were also discussed. One gain that was noted was that taking care of oral health can lead to improved quality of life, better nutrition, and improved physical and systemic health. Another gain is that innovations in materials and technology result in an easier delivery of care and provide better access to care. An example of this is teledentistry, which can take away some of the pains in terms of accessibility of oral health care for persons with disabilities. Finally, another gain that was discussed for this interest group was the progress being made toward inclusion. Improvements in awareness, acknowledgment, and acceptance, as reflected in recent changes to National Institutes of Health policies, are important gains for persons with disabilities. McNeil commented that there is still work to be done, but positive signs of change are happening now.

In discussing what it would take to achieve the top three gains while minimizing the mentioned pains, the breakout group leads noted three important aspects (Figure 3-4). McNeil reported on conversations from his breakout group where educators were being called upon to train students to be competent providers for persons with disabilities, and this would include didactic and experiential training. Additionally, payment plans for this type of work would be very important. He also suggested that there is a social shift in students and dental educators, and that educators are behind students in terms of their focus on social justice. Lastly, McNeil reported the view discussed in his breakout group that persons with disabilities and caregivers be involved in education to better train dental students and residents. People with disabilities use the statement "For us, with us, by us," to make sure they are included in decision making, education, and care to make things better for their group. To achieve this goal, said McNeil, it is important that there is collaboration of all professional groups, not just dental, but a broad array of medicine, behavioral, and social scientists as well, alongside persons with disabilities and caregivers who must be included as agents of change.

What will it take for educators and providers to achieve their top three gains while minimizing the pains?

- Educators to truly train students to be competent providers (time; comfort of educators). Didactic and experiential training. Payment element for providers and education of all providers (medical/dental/etc).
- Educators need to catch-up to students. Persons with disabilities and caregivers involved in education

Will it involve other stakeholder groups?

- Collaboration of all professional groups as well as persons with disabilities and caregivers.

FIGURE 3-4 Oral health value proposition for persons with disabilities.
SOURCE: Presentation by Marshall and McNeil, February 16, 2024.

Providers and Educators

The second breakout group discussed the value proposition model for interprofessional providers and educators. This breakout group was led by Jeffrey Stewart and Cynthia Lord. Lord explained that the group discussed several pain points for providers and listed three items as most important (Table 3-3a). One of these pain points is that providers are unable to change federal or state policies. There are no valid research data that a different model of providing oral health care in a medical setting would improve patient care, she said. This results in medical schools not being incentivized to teach oral health care. The second pain point discussed evolves around the siloed ways in which care is provided to patients. There is a need for more integration of dental care with medical care. Working together and understanding the benefits and patient needs are important for this, Lord noted. The third pain point involves issues with the system, including documentation, billing, and coding. Since these are conducted separately for medical and dental care, it increases the gap between the two, which led to a conversation about a need for integrated electronic health records for best patient outcomes, she said.

Lord then described the group's discussion about educators. Educators have two pain points, she said (Table 3-3b). While there are the Interprofessional Education Collaborative competencies and accreditation standards that require interprofessional work, the breakout group talked about how interprofessional education has "a long way to go" in integrating faculty

TABLE 3-3a Oral Health Value Proposition Pains for Providers

PAIN	RATIONALE
Inability to change federal/state policies: *No valid research data that a different model of providing oral health care in a medical setting would have an impact on patient care.*	Schools are not incentivized to teach oral health since there is currently no evidence it improves patient outcomes.
Siloed care: *Medical care and dental care gap; need to be geographically in the same place, working together, to understand patient needs.*	Need integrated medical/dental care for the best patient outcomes
Systems issue: *Documentation, billing, coding, etc. are separate for dental and medical, therefore increasing the gap.*	Need integrated electronic health record for the best patient outcomes

SOURCE: Presentation by Stewart and Lord on February 16, 2024.

TABLE 3-3b Oral Health Value Proposition Pains for Educators and Providers

PAIN	RATIONALE
Interprofessional education (IPE): *Although health professions' accreditation standards require IPE, it does not say how or how much should be taught among institutions.*	Schools are not integrated and very siloed; integration needs to start early in a student's educational process. IPE must be valued as a basic science and clinical medicine and should not be considered "optional."
Lack of basic education across professions: *Medical students are taught very little or no oral health. Specialists exist for a reason, but there is still a need for interprofessional collaboration.*	Need to understand how dental health affects rest of the body, despite your specialty.

SOURCE: Presentation by Stewart and Lord, February 16, 2024.

and processes in oral health. Schools are still very siloed in terms of medical and dental care education. To improve this, Lord commented, there is a need to start early in a student's educational process. Interprofessional education exists, but it is not standardized and should be more highly valued, like basic science and clinical medicine. These factors are important to ensure practitioners work together and maintain a patient-centered approach, Lord said.

Lord said the gains for providers and educators include the potential use of electronic health records (Table 3-4). Integrating dental records with

TABLE 3-4 Oral Health Value Proposition Gains for Educators and Providers

GAIN	RATIONALE
Electronic health record that integrates with the medical side (need to integrate education modules).	Could not communicate without it.
Students' desire to learn from each other.	Facilitates interprofessional collaboration.
Dental office can serve as a portal into the medical system (e.g., blood pressure).	Can facilitate entrance into the medical system when problems are identified.
Accreditation standards (interprofessional education, caring for patients with special needs, etc.)	Improves overall capabilities; can align with needs of institution

SOURCE: Presentation by Stewart and Lord, February 16, 2024.

medical records would be essential to allow for effective communication between the siloes. Another gain is that students have the desire to learn from each other, and this can facilitate interprofessional collaboration. Lord said that students care a lot about being efficient and sharing information. There is excitement from learners who, as noted in the group discussions, want more interprofessional collaborative opportunities. Additionally, dental offices can serve as portals into the medical system, she said, by providing screening and identifying problems detected during routine dental exams. Lord then commented that accreditation standards are essential. The standards exist now and include interprofessional work, but more can be done using accreditation as a building block on which to expand.

For educational gains, Lord called out the group's emphasis on interprofessional education to effectively care for persons with special needs. This, she said, can align with the needs of educational institutions, especially when it improves the overall capabilities of the institution.

In describing what it will take to achieve the gains while minimizing the pains, Lord summarized the group's conversation by saying it is important for dental professionals to interact with undergraduate students to help promote the field and relationships. Provider reimbursements are also key, she added, because without financing, there is no incentive for change. A collaborative spirit will go a long way to achieving interprofessional collaboration, which can be supported by minimizing competition among related specialties. Addressing scope-of-practice issues was also discussed by the group; it believed such issues require policy changes and input from other interest groups. More specifically, Lord said, professional associations can amplify what it takes to become a specialist, and policy makers can weigh in on the sorts of tests or procedures that can be run by oral versus medical health specialists. Lord added that if patients or persons with disabilities and their caretakers demand change, if they are convinced that oral health will improve their overall health, this group can work with providers and educators to push policy makers for what they feel is better care.

During the discussion, participants brought up additional pain points, including challenges to education integration caused by an already overloaded curriculum. Lord responded by saying that oral health is already included in topics in medical school as it is all connected; it does not require separate courses. Online participants also noted stress and burnout, particularly for students. Lord suggested that maybe there would be less of both if there was more interprofessional collaboration.

An oral health value proposition for educators and providers is presented in Figure 3-5.

What will it take for educators and providers to achieve their top three gains while minimizing the pains?

- Dental professionals should interact with undergrads, etc. (do it EARLY) to help promote the field and relationships between them.
- Provider reimbursements – without this, there is no incentive. Even if health professions students were taught the importance of working interprofessionally, it will depend on the environment/culture they are working in whether it happens in clinical practice.
- Need collaborative spirit and not competition between related specialties
- Scope of practice – need to change and expand (e.g., vaccine delivery). Need policy changes. Expand scope of ability AND scope of attitude!

Will it involve other stakeholder groups? YES

- Professional associations that recommend what it takes to be a specialist.
- Policymakers in each state – dictates what you can test for, etc.
- Patients – if they are convinced oral health is better for their health, they will push for it.
- Recenter on the patient/person.

FIGURE 3-5 Oral health value proposition for educators and providers.
SOURCE: Presentation by Stewart and Lord, February 16, 2024.

Payers and Policy Makers

The third breakout group, led by Marko Vujicic and Donna M. Hallas, discussed the pains and gains (Tables 3-5 and 3-6) for a potential oral value proposition for the payers and policy makers interest group. Vujicic explained that the pain points discussed in the breakout group included existing payment models. First, current incentive structures are reinforcing disease treatment rather than rewarding health, and these structures are a major driver of provider behavior, he said. This is true for both the public insurance programs and the private insurance programs. Second, there is a lack of usable, actionable, and integrated data and information. This includes a lack of medical and dental health information in the same health record, patient-reported outcomes, and identifying patients with disabilities. In particular, data that are usable and actionable are missing. Third, clinical guidelines can facilitate policy changes, but there is currently a lack of prescriptive directives. For instance, if the system were to move toward one that promotes health wellness, focusing on prevention, is the science there to direct how to keep a patient free of caries, Vujicic asked. Not enough protocols might exist right now to answer this question.

Potential gains discussed by the interest group included cost savings. It is essential that a financial return on investment be provided for the enhancement of oral health, Vujicic said. This would not only include the health care cost savings, but also factors such as better employment and quality of life. Another possible gain is better care. Vujicic noted that this is a slow movement in the U.S. health care system. There is movement of the systems toward a focus on outcomes and better quality of care. The final

TABLE 3-5 Oral Health Value Proposition Pains for Payers and Policy Makers

PAIN	RATIONALE
Payment Models: *Incentive structures are simply reinforcing treating disease rather than rewarding health (both in private and public insurance).*	Major driver of provider behavior.
Data: *Lack of usable, actionable, and integrated data, including patient-reported outcomes, and identifying with disabilities.*	No data = no info.
Clinical Guidelines: *Guidelines are needed to change policy (e.g., guidelines for diabetes management to include dental screenings).*	As much as "doing the right thing" is touted, prescriptive directives are needed.

SOURCE: Presentation by Vujicic and Hallas, February 16, 2024.

TABLE 3-6 Oral Health Value Proposition Gains for Payers and Policy Makers

GAIN	RATIONALE
Cost savings	Fiscal impacts rule. It is important to provide a financial return on investment to enhanced oral health in terms of health care cost savings, as well as better employment and better life.
Better care	With the system moving toward a focus on outcomes, better health is a key value.
Equity	Finally being recognized as a priority within health care policy in the United States, especially within public insurance programs.

SOURCE: Presentation by Vujicic and Hallas, February 16, 2024.

gain his group discussed was a commitment to solutions related to equity, and the recognition of equity as a priority within U.S. health care policy. This is particularly true within public insurance programs, Vujicic added. Like the other interest group reports, his group felt that to achieve these gains, while reducing the pains, collaboration with all other interest groups would be essential (Figure 3-6).

What will it take for payers & policy makers to achieve their top three gains while minimizing the pains?

> Private Insurance – market/sales driven; It needs to sell. Unless dental benefits all of a sudden become much more regulated, this action will only come through $.

> Public Insurance - regulate comprehensive coverage in public programs.

> Regulators – regulate interoperability, incentivize harmonization of records

Will it involve other stakeholder groups?

Yes

FIGURE 3-6 Oral health value proposition for payers and policy makers.
SOURCE: Presentation by Vujicic and Hallas, February 16, 2024.

4

Whole Health Through Oral Health

BOX 4-1
Key Points Made by Individual Speakers*

- School-based health centers can provide holistic health services for students, staff, and community members. (Hall)
- Providing training for mental health care professionals in Zimbabwe raised community awareness of the oral health needs of patients with mental health conditions. (Matanhire and Murembwe-Machingauta)
- Nurse training and an oral health information card included with an infant's vaccination card was an effective way to decrease the prevalence of cavities in Peru. (Villena)
- Students form interprofessional teams and are connected with an individual or family participant in the community ... to collaborate with them to promote oral and overall health and well-being. (Ensz)
- Rather than expecting patients to come in and get the care, the health care team takes the initiative and finds the patients. (Devalia)

*This list is the rapporteurs' summary of points made by the individual speakers identified, and the statements have not been endorsed or verified by the National Academies of Sciences, Engineering, and Medicine. They are not intended to reflect a consensus among workshop participants.

A session on Whole Health through oral health was introduced by Robert Weyant. He opened by emphasizing the importance of exploring connections between oral health and overall health and well-being. Poor oral health is a gateway to systemic illness, he said, affecting chronic illnesses and mental well-being. Oral health is not an isolated domain but an integral part of a person's entire being, extending far beyond the dental chair into the realm of comprehensive health and wellness. He described the session as a journey around the globe starting first with a presentation about school-based holistic clinics in rural Oregon, then traveling to Zimbabwe, Peru, and Britain, before returning back to the United States for a virtual presentation from Florida. Together, these presentations provide a unique narrative that transcends borders and disciplines and emphasizes the integral role that oral health plays in achieving Whole Health. He introduced the speakers by inviting the audience "to engage in this transformative journey with our distinguished speakers and contribute to the global dialogue and the inseparable connection between oral health and comprehensive well-being."

SCHOOL-BASED HEALTH CENTERS

Karen Hall, the oral health integration manager of Capitol Dental Care in Oregon, shared data about school-based health centers that provide holistic health services for students, staff, and community members. In the United States, there are 3,900 school-based health centers, said Hall, and in 2022, a survey was performed on 40 percent of the centers in the United States (School-Based Health Alliance, 2023). Most of these centers are located onsite at an elementary, middle, or high school. Many school-based centers bring in mobile clinics to provide additional services, such as dental or vision care. Each provider at the center bills separately and has different referral pathways to specialists to get care outside of the center.

Hall explained this concept by using one center as an example: the Central Health and Wellness Center. This school-based center provides comprehensive care, including dental, behavioral health, mental health, and primary care. Providers often screen patients for services outside of their area of expertise; for example, the medical provider screens for dental needs and will make the necessary referral if an intervention is indicated. Staff have identified benefits to working at the center, including providing wraparound services for patients to receive holistic care, which has resulted in shared learning by staff and lower staff turnover rates. Further, Hall said, family members can see different providers during the same appointment visit, saving them time and making it easier to coordinate with work and school. Hall noted that approximately 1,266 unique patients were served in 2023 at the wellness center for a total of over 2,100 visits. Roughly half of the patients were community members, and 30 percent were served by more than one provider, she said.

A member of the audience asked Hall if families have to opt in for each of these services. Hall answered saying that patients are required to provide signed consent for each of the services. This led Weyant to ask how funding is secured for the centers. Hall said that each entity has its own funding mechanisms and sees mainly patients from the Medicaid population. Overall, this has been a sustainable way of funding the centers.

ORAL HEALTH PROMOTION AND CARE
FOR PATIENTS WITH MENTAL HEALTH
CONDITIONS IN ZIMBABWE

Cleopatra Matanhire, Department of Oral Health, University of Zimbabwe, and director of the Oral Ling Axis Trust, and Kudzai Murembwe-Machingauta, training coordinator at Oral Ling Axis Trust and technical lead for Covid Go at OPHID at the Africa University Zimbabwe, described the situation in Zimbabwe and outlined their work in creating a basic package of oral health promotion and care for patients with mental health conditions. The duo, from medicine and dentistry, explained that the health care system in Zimbabwe is constrained in terms of money and human resources. The Ministry of Health and Childcare Services in Zimbabwe provides free services and dental care for people living with mental health conditions. Matanhire and Murembwe-Machingauta provided training for mental health care professionals to raise community awareness of the oral health and dental treatment needs of these patients. They discussed the situation at an institute for mental health where many mental health providers work, but the institute had only one dental technician, who was underused. The pair provided interprofessional training so other providers could conduct simple oral exams, refer patients to dental providers when needed, and raise alarms when patients reported being in pain. This change in approach brought providers together, helping them to find new ways to collaborate.

In the future, Matanhire and Murembwe-Machingauta plan to take their efforts into communities to engage caregivers and work with churches and places where they believe they can have a positive impact. However, the economic situation in Zimbabwe has led to a shortage of basic oral hygiene aids, said Matanhire. This led them to a new plan where they will go back to more traditional oral medicines readily available in the environment to overcome this obstacle while also studying the value of these traditional medicines for oral health. Further, the medical–dental team intends to expand into the private sector to help make treatments more accessible and bring training to a virtual platform to allow and expand their reach beyond the provinces in which they currently work. Overall, their goal is to influence policy and to ensure that training for mental and oral health professionals is adequate to cater to the needs of vulnerable populations.

Before leaving the stage, Weyant asked Matanhire and Murembwe-Machingauta whether dental providers in Zimbabwe also ever perform mental health assessments. Matanhire responded that dental providers are trained in Zimbabwe together with medical colleagues in all courses and rotations. To a certain extent, she said, there is already a level of knowledge there to facilitate the possibility.

INTEGRATING ORAL HEALTH INTO GENERAL HEALTH AT INFANCY

Rita S. Villena, chair of the Pediatric Dentistry Department at the University San Martin de Porres in Peru, spoke next. She discussed a program initiated in Peru, where there is a high percentage of early childhood caries in the first 36 months of life, in part because of inequalities in the country with access to care. Villena implemented a new initiative as part of the already existing mother and child program, which is a mandatory and easy-to-access program that includes health checks and vaccinations. For this program, a protocol was created to integrate oral health into general health, working with nurses in charge of the program. The nurses received training, after which a study was performed. Villena said the study showed that education and the use of an oral health information and record card included with the vaccination card was an effective way to decrease the prevalence of cavities. Furthermore, in the study group, there were no pulp-involvement lesions and therefore no one required more invasive treatments. The study showed that these effects resulted in lower costs. Villena said the oral health information card was essential as a tool to connect the nurses in the program with the dentist. Villena argued that installing good habits "during infancy" is easier than changing bad habits at later ages.

Weyant asked if Villena was planning to scale her educational intervention, and if so, how she plans to undertake the expansion. Villena said that having established the scientific support for the initiative, she and her colleagues do plan to expand the program. Recently, the idea was proposed to the Ministry of Health so, if approved, Villena is hopeful she will be able to offer the program to the whole country. A follow-up question asked Villena what barriers she thinks she will need to overcome, particularly when moving the initiative from private to public organizations. Villena responded that a key barrier to scaling up the program will be training the workforce, which includes training dentists to treat infants. Weyant added that such training would have to be ongoing as turnover of staff occurs.

COMMUNITY-BASED OUTREACH EDUCATION IN FLORIDA

The next to present was Olga S. Ensz, director of community-based outreach at the University of Florida. She discussed the Putting Families First service learning experience at the University of Florida that has been in place for 25 years. In this program, students form interprofessional teams and are connected with an individual or family member in the community. This experience allows students from different backgrounds to come together and become immersed in a community member's life outside of a clinical setting, to recognize the unique challenges and social determinants the community member may face, and to collaborate with them to promote their oral and overall health and well-being, Ensz said.

The program includes students from dentistry, medicine, nursing, pharmacy, public health and health professions, and veterinary medicine. The goal of the project is to develop a collaborative person-centered health promotion project. Specifically, it aims to have students understand how social, cultural, economic, and political determinants affect individual, animal, and population health. Further, Ensz said, the program advocates recognizing the importance of interprofessional collaboration in health care, because once students understand how to work interprofessionally, they will be ready to enter the workforce as members of a collaborative practice team.

In the discussion with the audience, a participant asked whether there are data to say if the program improves patient outcomes. Ensz answered that it is unclear whether the program affects health outcomes of the community members participating as that is not measured. However, it is known that participants develop a greater awareness of resources that are available to them and they enhance their medical knowledge. Another audience member asked if there were data on whether students continued this type of interprofessional collaboration later in their careers. Ensz explained that currently no data are captured as to whether this program enhances interprofessional collaboration in practice after education.

MINI MOUTH CARE MATTERS IN ENGLAND

Urshla Devalia, consultant pediatric dentist at Eastman Dental Hospital at UCLH (London) and national lead for Mini Mouth Care Matters, was the final speaker of this session. She began her presentation saying that in England there are major issues in the health care system with dental services where the funding system does not incentivize prevention care. This results in many children and young people needing anesthetic treatment for teeth to be removed. In the UK, the British Society of Pediatric Dentistry has coordinated with the Royal College of Pediatrics and Child Health to provide a definition of dental neglect. This is defined as the persistent failure to meet a child's basic oral health needs, likely to result in serious impairments of a child's oral or general health or development.

Devalia described the oral health situation as being "in the worst crisis the nation has seen in the last 75 years, according to research conducted by the Nuffield Trust" (Williams et al., 2023a). While the cause of the crisis is multifactorial, stemming mainly from lack of funding and too few oral health providers serving in the National Health Services, the situation and personal experiences as a pediatric dentist motivated Devalia and her colleagues to start a program in the UK called Mini Mouth Care Matters (Mini MCM). The program was launched in 2019 and focused on "making every contact count." Training was delivered to make sure that medical and allied health care professionals were provided with the knowledge, skills, and tools to recognize what healthy and unhealthy mouths look like.

The project started in the inpatient setting and was later expanded. For this program a hospital guide and a suite of online course materials were developed. Devalia said that all practitioners were trained to look into the mouth and, using the Mini MCM mouth care assessment tool, identify those children and young people with unmet dental needs and direct them to appropriate services. With the health care team taking the oral health advice and prevention to the patients, they can reinforce prevention messages and seek out those who require care, as opposed to those attending dental clinics in an emergency situation.

More recently, Devalia worked with care providers for children and young people with special needs to "work with those groups who don't necessarily have a voice to see what matters to them to tailor the resources appropriately." She presented some examples of the projects that aimed to improve the situation for those with disabilities. A dental passport was developed that each patient carries with them, stating their likes, dislikes, and what they want to avoid when coming into the dental clinic to help those with sensory needs. Her team also created information for families to help them cope with children who might have sensory challenges with toothbrushing, and a dental pain communication chart was created for nonverbal patients.

Devalia described how she used all of the resources in a remote setting. Teledentistry enables assessments to be performed with a parent or caregiver present who the child is comfortable with. The parent or caregiver can then discuss the child's situation with a dentist who can determine where the child needs to be seen to ensure dental interventions take place in an appropriate setting for that child or young person. When asked if there was any additional reimbursement for the health providers doing the mouth assessments, Devalia noted that in the British system this is not an issue as everybody is paid their salary within a hospital setting, so there is no need for additional funding for a project like this. Hall then asked if dentistry is also privatized in the UK. Devalia responded that because dentistry is free for children under 16 years of age, and up to 18 years for those in full-time education, privatized pediatric dentistry is not common.

An audience member noted that the United States and the UK spend substantial amounts of funding and health care resources on trying to treat tooth decay in primary teeth in children under the age of 6 years, and then the rest of their lives it seems to become scarce. While not disagreeing, Devalia did comment that the wider picture and social determinants of health should be considered, "Inequalities are common, and teeth are often the collateral damage," she said.

5

Fitting the Value Proposition into the Larger Picture

BOX 5-1
Key Points Made by Individual Speakers*

- Equitable oral health services is not really about equal access ... but about fairness. (Helgeson)
- A Whole Health home for persons with disabilities offers comprehensive care, holistic support, person-centered care, preventive care, improved quality of life, empowerment and self-advocacy, reduced health disparities, and enhanced care coordination. (Glick)

*This list is the rapporteurs' summary of points made by the individual speakers identified, and the statements have not been endorsed or verified by the National Academies of Sciences, Engineering, and Medicine. They are not intended to reflect a consensus among workshop participants.

Teresa Marshall, professor at the Department of Preventive and Community Dentistry at the University of Iowa, opened the session by reminding the audience of the following:

Up until now, we have been discussing what a value proposition is and how we might consider building such a proposition for persons with disabilities so all interest groups see value in holistic oral health promotion and disease prevention in persons with disabilities.

53

Building on that notion, Marshall said the focus for this session would be on where the value proposition might be applied by hearing from two presenters. The first focused on equity, and the second looked at a Whole Health home for oral health.

ORAL HEALTH EQUITY

Michael Helgeson is the chief executive officer at Apple Tree Dental. He discussed what oral health equity is and why it is essential, how Apple Tree helps create more equitable health care systems, and how policy makers can help to make care more equitable by funding pilot projects on new value-based care systems. Equitable oral health services is not really about equal access, he explained, but about fairness (see Figure 5-1). This is not the same thing for everyone. It requires tailored work and the recognition of the diverse oral health needs of individual patients and communities. He noted that providers must learn from the patient advocates and each other to provide equitable care. This will require interprofessional teams to collaborate in a variety of settings. Helgeson then moved one step further and explained that beyond equity, there is justice (see Figure 5-1), and for him, oral health justice is the goal. At Apple Tree Dental, he and his colleagues aim to remove the systemic barriers to create just and equitable oral health delivery systems.

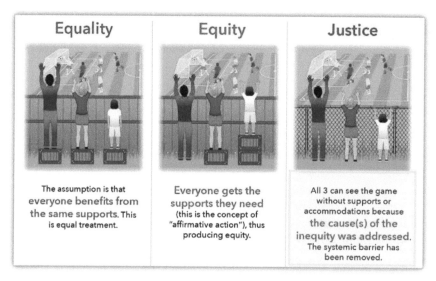

FIGURE 5-1 The difference between equality, equity, and justice in health care. SOURCE: Helgeson presentation, February 16, 2024. Reprinted with kind permission from agentsofgood.org.

In terms of payers, Helgeson feels that Medicaid, Medicare, and other public programs must provide equitable oral health benefits. This would mean different benefits for different groups. Further, on the side of the educators, increased interprofessional education in real-life clinical care settings would help achieve oral health justice. Lastly, he believes that communities must collaborate to remove barriers to health so the goal of oral health justice can be achieved.

Apple Tree Dental is a nonprofit organization, with a mission to overcome barriers to good oral health and a vision to foster partnerships that create healthy communities, Helgeson said. Located in Minnesota, the nonprofit has nine centers for dental health, and year-round collaborations with over 150 organizations, including Head Start centers, group homes, long-term care facilities, and mental health campuses. Some of these centers are integrated within hospitals and medical primary care. In these centers, he said, team members work together in interprofessional groups, with experts in geriatrics, pediatrics, dental, and public health. The centers are also engaged in system change with educational programs and public policy programs. According to Helgeson, partnering with community leaders helps the team design and launch local programs, which is their model of growth. This makes it driven by community interest.

The interprofessional work environment is designed to integrate dental care into health homes. As an example, Helgeson discussed the Rochester Center. The Rochester community was activated by Dr. Sarah Crane, a geriatrician at the Mayo Clinic, who had seen the results of neglect of patients in nursing homes. She helped lead the fundraising effort to establish an elder care program in Rochester. This is set up with mobile units and can accommodate people in wheelchairs and other medical aid tools. The units have all the gear that is found in a regular dental office, and services provided include fillings, extractions, root canals, and dentures. The clinical team works with the nurses at the nursing home, and post-op checkups can be performed in the afternoon in the resident's own room after receiving surgery in the morning, he said.

A few years later, in 2014, the Rochester Center was launched, which is based across the street from the Mayo Clinic. This center is now one of the major sources of critical-access dental care for all patients in that area, and it provides both mobile and hub services.

According to Helgeson, the key to success is being driven by passionate local leaders and being governed by an interprofessional board. Programs are designed with feasibility studies and business planning, are broadly supported by the community, and are designed for long-term sustainability. Interprofessional education experiences are possible in this setting, he said. Apple Tree Dental has agreements with educational institutions to host student rotations, a residency program, and a high school program, which is a career equity program.

Helgeson then detailed what value-based care entails. It requires building a system that pays for patient health outcomes and can lead to a more just and equitable health care system. He suggested that focusing on the oral health of people with disabilities and seniors has the greatest potential as a place to start. Because the total health care costs for these groups are highest, the likely economic benefit and quality-of-life advantage for these populations will provide the highest return on investment.

To achieve the sort of equitable system Helgeson envisions, one would have to start with the current system, he said, given that Medicaid dental benefits are not at present equitable. Helgeson suggested creating a special needs dental benefit and collaborating with early adopters to accelerate the process. To determine the success of the program, he said it is essential to measure things that matter. A publication on dental patient-reported outcomes measurement described four dimensions to patient oral health outcomes: oral function, orofacial pain, orofacial appearance (aesthetic), and psychosocial impact. Helgeson explained that these four dimensions can be measured using a simple questionnaire such as the OHIP-5 (John, 2022). The scored questionnaire indicates to the provider if there are problems within any of the domains and where a person is "in terms of the impact of oral health on their life," he said. "In the end," he said, "the goal is to move from being not healthy to being healthy."

Helgeson provided an overview of two pilot models with early adopters. The first is a project in which Apple Tree collaborates with a health plan in Minnesota. They are creating an integrated care coordination system and using the OHIP-5 to measure what counts, as well as creating new whole-health pathways using telehealth and other techniques. The second pilot is to determine how to scale up nonprofit organizations such as Apple Tree more rapidly. At Apple Tree, Helgeson and his colleagues have developed a model that uses program-related investment loans and other investments that can be made by health plans to expand their oral health provider network and generate a return on investment.

In the discussion that followed, an audience member from Penn Dental Medicine shared that the Apple Tree model was studied to better understand how to create equity in dental practices in the future, which was then integrated into the local and global public health course for 1st-year students. Another audience member asked what the key factor was to get launched when this idea was first conceived. Helgeson replied that the most important thing to get started is planning. He said that each new project gets launched with a feasibility study, which involves geographically defining the area of concern, identifying all needs, identifying the interest groups in a community, meeting with them, asking what they want to do, and then designing something that meets their needs. Next, a business plan is developed with an economic model for sustainability; it cannot be something that depends on ongoing operating grants. The core activities must pay for themselves, Helgeson said.

Another audience member asked Helgeson what would be "the thing" he would fix if he had a magic wand. Helgeson responded that he would make special care dental benefits in Medicaid. The system does not fit the requirements of children, people with disabilities, or seniors, he said. These people need a mix of services that are not covered and are not covered in the Code on Dental Procedures and Nomenclature (CDT). It could start with CDT codes to make it easier to scale up these kinds of services. This can be done while value-based care is being built, which flows through health plans, allowing multitasking, Helgeson said. Finally, Betsy Lee White commented that there are models that work, but understanding the community is key to this. Therefore, she suggested that when looking at a systems change, to consider what the best of these models are and work together in collaboration.

Mark Wolff commented that he agrees with Helgeson on compensation and taking people with disabilities out of the Medicaid system, which was designed for indigent individuals. Wolff also noted that he thinks it should be a national policy because people with disabilities get treated differently in different states. He further noted the "obligation we have" to find an equitable health solution. Helgeson agreed with these comments and said that he thinks special needs dental benefits can be provided. He said that Medicaid has data on disabilities, and existing classifications can be used, so there would be no prior authorization barriers and people with various conditions would be eligible for certain additional benefits.

Lastly, an online participant asked about the source of funding for the feasibility studies and needs assessments in the initial planning phases. Helgeson responded by saying that it is usually funded in collaboration with the local community. Referring to a previous comment by Glassman, he said, "The money is there. It's just a matter of getting the money in the right buckets where it is well spent."

A WHOLE ORAL HEALTH HOME

Michael Glick, executive director of the Center for Integrative Global Oral Health and Fields-Rayant professor at Penn Dental Medicine, presented his perspective on a Whole Health home for oral health. He began by telling the audience that for collaboration to happen, the various collaborators need to speak the same language and share the same definitions. For this reason, Glick went through a series of definitions in order to frame what is meant by *whole-person health*.

Last year, he said, the National Academies of Science, Engineering, and Medicine published a consensus study report on achieving Whole Health (NASEM, 2023). This report described Whole Health as physical, behavioral, spiritual, and socioeconomic well-being, as defined by individuals, families, and communities. Whole Health care is an interprofessional, team-based approach, anchored in trusted relationships to promote well-being, prevent disease, and restore health. A Whole Health approach, he said, requires changing the health care conversation from "What is wrong with you?" to "What matters to you?" Glick noted that this goes back to many of the topics discussed at this workshop, such as talking about the health and well-being of communities, not of individuals only. Restoring health goes beyond just taking care of disease, he said. It aligns with a person's life, mission, aspiration, and purpose.

Glick noted that the FDI World Dental Federation came up with a definition of oral health that was approved in 2016 by the World Dental Parliament, which represents over a million dentists in the world (Glick, 2016). This definition states that oral health is multifaceted and includes the ability to speak, smile, smell, taste, touch, chew, swallow, and convey emotions through facial expression with confidence and without pain, discomfort, and disease of the craniofacial complex. Glick then discussed how these aspects of the definition can be studied and measured. Creating a value system would facilitate the measurement and allow for reflections on the physiological, social, and psychological attributes that are essential for a good quality of life, which is influenced by an individual's changing experiences, perceptions, expectations, and ability to adapt to circumstances throughout their lifespan.

Next, Glick discussed a framework, presented in Figure 5-2, pointing out the three different domains. The disease and conditions form the top, and on the bottom there are physiological function and psychosocial function or status. Additionally, there are driving determinants and moderating factors. These are very important for health, Glick said. Driving determinants are elements such as genetic biological factors, social and economic factors, and social support networks. These are often the root causes or fundamental forces that shape the outcome. They are key factors that need to be addressed to get to overall oral health, Glick explained. Moderating factors are factors that influence the strength or the direction of the relationship between two other variables. These do not directly cause the outcome but rather modify the relationship between the driving determinants and the outcomes. Moderating factors include age, culture, income, experience, expectation, and adaptability. Such factors are difficult to measure in studies, he said.

Glick then went back to his earlier comments on the importance of speaking the same language. While many are talking about multidisciplinary

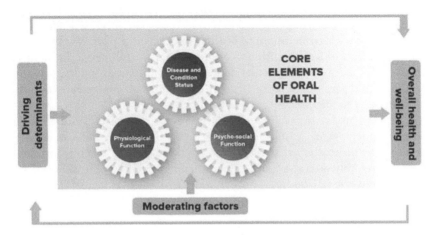

FIGURE 5-2 A framework for the definition of oral health.
SOURCE: Glick presentation, February 16, 2024. Reprinted from Glick et al., 2016. A new definition for oral health developed by the FDI World Dental Federation opens the door to a universal definition of oral health. *The Journal of the American Dental Association* 147(12):915-917, with permission from the American Dental Association.

(i.e., professions working side by side) and interdisciplinary (i.e., professions working toward a common goal), there is also a need to talk about transdisciplinary, he said. Transdisciplinary means that boundaries between and beyond disciplines are transcended, and knowledge and perspective from different scientific disciplines and nonscientific sources are integrated (Choi and Pak, 2006). Transdisciplinary education and care can include things like urban planning, transportation, law, education, and sociology. Glick suggested starting to look at transdisciplinary when it comes to Whole Health and where to go next.

A Whole Health home, Glick said, is a collaborative transdisciplinary preventive care model where people's values, or issues that are important to them, take center stage with goals for disease prevention, improved health outcomes, and well-being through the life course. A Whole Health home for persons with disabilities offers comprehensive care, holistic support, person-centered care, preventive care, improved quality of life, empowerment and self-advocacy, reduced health disparities, and enhanced care coordination. Therefore, embracing the Whole Health concept or home concept represents a transformative step toward a more integrated person-centered health care system that promises improved outcomes and enhanced well-being for individuals and communities.

To achieve this, Glick suggested that a health care system could prioritize a transdisciplinary coordinated care model, increased awareness, engagement with contemporary health concepts and partners, improving the integration of health within overall health and well-being. In addition, there could be recognition, understanding, and addressing equity, diversity, and inclusion across different marginalized and disadvantaged communities throughout the life course.

The discussion following Glick's presentation started with an audience member asking a question drawn from the adage, "Home is where you can go no matter what time it is." Is there a place where someone in pain can reliably go for definitive care when it is evening or a weekend and, for example, the person has a broken tooth? Might that sort of on-demand care be incorporated into the whole home concept? Glick replied that his concept of a Whole Health home is not so much a physical space but the integration of different services. For instance, a community member could help someone in need of dental care or preventive services by connecting that person to an appropriate health system for care. An online participant asked whether one of the linkages in a transdisciplinary model between different areas could be libraries or sources of information, data management, and mining. Would the conduits and managers be the librarians and information professionals? Glick replied that librarians could indeed help with this.

A representative from Arc of Philadelphia commented on the importance of thinking about how to integrate the disability service system with health care delivery, as these systems are more aware of how somebody with intellectual disabilities can use community-based services around the clock. Disability services are often perceived as separate from health care delivery, and they are underfunded. These services often must overcome the negative effects of the social determinants of health, he said.

John Kemp commented that it is imperative that schools and other groups become part of the advocacy program that extends the lifespan and is part of the disability movement and vice versa. It is important to expand connections so all can advocate together for improved transportation systems, personal care, attendance services, home health aides, and delivering services in the home and not just in the community itself. It is important to provide services to people where the people are, he said. Helen Lee remarked that the comment on transdisciplinary collaboration sparked a thought that, during the workshop, there was a discussion on how to integrate the world and the human experience into oral health, but what if this were flipped? In this case, the answer would be pushed into other aspects of the human experience that have nothing directly to do with health— bringing in urban planning, for example—as ways to push the agenda forward. Glick supported such "out of the box" thinking and encouraged engagement across sectors for continued learning from and with others.

A participant asked whether there are programs for students on this Whole Health approach in terms of an interdisciplinary or transdisciplinary method of treating patients. Mark Wolff, dean of Penn Dental Medicine, responded that areas at the school were even pushing to include veterinary medicine in these discussions. There are multiple health programs within the school, and the best example, he said, is the newest venture, which will have an integrated health record and dental record that is bidirectional. Additionally, there is a recently opened hospital and federally qualified health center outpatient clinic where the plan is to have students work with public health hygienists and medical providers. Glick added that there is also a course about critical thinking, which is about how to evaluate data and research and how to understand and interpret it. This is an important step to moving the Whole Health approach forward, he said.

Natalia Chalmers noted that while integration has been discussed for a long time, there are few examples of it being seamlessly and successfully implemented. Because of the flexibility states have under Medicaid to decide what dental services are covered for adults, there is geographic variation. The encouraging news, she said, is that the number of states offering only emergency adult dental services is decreasing.

Glassman shared that his colleagues in California have examples of integrating and using home-based and community-based services for people with disabilities. The project is called Shortening-the-line, which aims to shorten the waiting lines for dental services in hospital operating rooms, in which care is brought into places where people are receiving services through social service systems in group homes and day programs (Williams et al., 2023b). This project is now finished, and Glassman predicts they will be able to shorten the line by 50 percent, as fewer people will be needing general anesthesia for dental care.

A VALUE PROPOSITION REVISITED

The final session of the workshop provided participants an opportunity to discuss how the different interest groups might consider implementing any of the ideas brought forward during the workshop. Berman introduced the session and asked participants to think about solutions in terms of "will it solve a real problem and bring some innovation and creativity." He also encouraged the audience to think out of the box. Instead of thinking about how to get the patient to the health system, he suggested, it might be worth considering how the health system can get to the patient; think about not only patients in health care but also things such as housing, work, and lifestyle.

Berman primed the audience, stating that the idea of the brainstorming session is to create a value proposition or something that has not been done before and meets the needs of all the interest groups. He reflected on some statements made about the problems individuals with disabilities face and what is not working well for them now. The question is how to incorporate something into a pilot project that would maybe be a technology, a service, a product, or maybe all of these. A good way to succinctly convey an idea is to come up with a name for the idea and a brief elevator speech, in which the idea is described. The short speech would emphasize what is special or different about the idea, and what problem is being solved and for whom.

An interactive session followed with all participants, both those at the meeting and those online. Using an online system, participants were asked to come up with keywords for a title of a pilot study for the value proposition. Using an online system, a word cloud was formed in real time while participants typed in and submitted their text (Figure 5-3). The main words that popped up were *transdisciplinary, disparities, interprofessional, equity, EverySystemEveryone, integration, interdisciplinary, well-being, whole person, value,* and *justice.*

OPEN DISCUSSION

In a final roundtable discussion led by Bruce Doll, workshop participants were given free reign to share anything discussed or not discussed at the workshop that could include key lessons from the workshop and ideas for the future. Doll asked participants to think about issues from their own personal perspectives that may have been shaped by the workshop's sessions—were there any surprises and did anyone's views change?

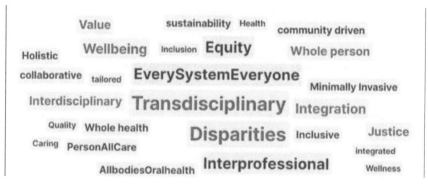

FIGURE 5-3 Value proposition word cloud.
SOURCE: Berman presentation, February 16, 2024.

System Change

An audience member raised his hand to say that this workshop made him realize how much work there is to be done in fixing the oral health care system. He suggested expressing their concerns through voting; otherwise, the politicians will not hear the voices of those who need to be heard.

Paul Glassman brought up his desire to bring dental care and preventive services into the community where people live. It is important to think more expansively about dental care, and only by changing delivery systems can value be changed. This includes integrating systems—not just medical systems, said Glassman, but also social and educational systems. There are examples of these in practice now, and they are growing, so increasing the focus on systems can fundamentally change the way people think about producing oral health for populations.

Berman asked Glassman if he thinks this can be done without increases in budgets. Glassman replied that it is absolutely possible, and, as he had mentioned earlier, it is a bucket problem. If the number of people with disabilities who are waiting for dental care under general anesthesia could be cut in half by providing care through a community desensitization model—such as receiving early intervention and prevention services in community locations—the total cost of care would be much lower. Using this model, money could be saved, he said. However, the problem is with the accounting systems, because it is not well recognized that such programs could lower the number of patients hospitalized and that it is worth spending some extra money on community-based services. These services and the funding for them comes from different buckets, and there are silos in the accounting system. So, Glassman argued, there is plenty of money in the system, but there is a need to think about spending it differently so cost-effective, person-centered care can be provided.

Marko Vujicic further discussed the question of whether enough money is in the system and whether prevention indeed leads to cost savings and restorations downstream. He said that the research seems to provide mixed results. Glassman answered that indeed, there is not enough research and convincing evidence on this, and it is difficult to study. However, he argued, there are data that point in this direction. For example, Glassman described a 6-year study he and colleagues performed in which dental hygienists worked in schools, using only minimally invasive procedures such as fluoride varnish and silver diamine fluoride. They were able to maintain the dental health of 80 percent of the children without needing to go to a dental office. The cost of running the program was approximately one-third of the cost of performing these procedures at a dental office, he said. Glassman noted that it may need to be framed differently and that prevention does not necessarily need to happen in a dental office to allow for cost savings. Vujicic agreed, as studies seem not to show that preventive dental care in offices provides a long-term return on investment, but delivering this care in the community or in schools creates several cost savings. However, he said, the problem is that these are not funded from the same pool of funds.

Urshla Devalia followed up by saying that prevention was not discussed enough during this meeting. She said there is an initiative called Child Smile based in Scotland that has shown a positive return on investment and demonstrated decreases in decayed, missing teeth caused by caries, and fewer filled teeth for children who were in a supervised toothbrushing program. This is a government-funded initiative. Devalia noted that whatever the solution, it would have to be a two-prong approach including accessibility and prevention. Reasonable adjustments, she felt, make sure the services get to those in the greatest need such as refugees, and those living in under-served communities. Devalia emphasized that prevention should be part of a transdisciplinary approach, not just through schoolteachers. Helen Lee commented that active prevention treatments work for some but not all people. Disease will always persist, she said, so from her perspective she would like to see more focus on overall health promotion.

John Garrett Picard from Pacific Dental Services said their foundation helps patients with special needs in Arizona. Most of these patients have some form of insurance, so insurance payers are integral to the discussion. There is a need for public service announcements (PSAs) to highlight the importance of oral health and well-being. He said that little effort has been put into ensuring that dental disease and periodontal disease are prevented. One could think of it like a tobacco cessation program, which could be cavity and periodontal cessation that uses PSAs to reach all people across the spectrum to prevent gum disease from happening. That, he felt, would be helpful for making a societal shift. In addition, an audience member suggested acknowledging the social determinants of health when discussing prevention. This would require breaking out of professional silos and engaging with others across professions and sectors. She said this workshop was a step in that direction.

Michael Glick noted that despite education on how to prevent dental disease, 45 percent of the world population has dental disease, so education is not working well. He also believes that patient expectations could be altered so that many do not see dental caries or oral disease as a natural process. Glick admitted that he does not know how to reach patients with this message, but he raised it as a behavioral issue that could be addressed inter- or transdisciplinarily. Rita Villena commented that for her oral health program in Peru, creating a link between professionals was helpful, and they did so using an oral health record card. A tool for working inter-professionally, such as this oral health record card, she thought could help improve oral health collaborations. These collaborative tools could also facilitate interactions with behavioral specialists.

Teresa Marshall wondered whether oral disease might be thought of in a similar manner as other chronic diseases, such as obesity and diabetes. Prevention starts in utero or even before pregnancy, she said. There is too much focus on sugars without encouraging an overall healthy diet. She underscored the importance of prevention in avoiding dental disease and other chronic health conditions. Robert Weyant agreed with this but added that complete oral disease prevention is difficult at the individual level and not possible at the population level. One could lower the percentage by interventions such as fluoride, he said, but there are many related factors that would have to be managed that are beyond the patient's or dentist's control. He also commented on the lack of evidence showing the value of prevention. Where there is evidence to suggest practices are not efficacious, those are the things that should be stopped.

Betsy Lee White joined the discussion to say that participants of the workshop do not have to wait for a report to be published to start initiating change. She challenged the group to figure out how to come together, stop having the discussion, and move forward. An online participant supported White's advocacy and added that it is important to realize that changing general population views on oral health promotion and prevention of oral disease starts with the participants here. The first step is to change the professional perspective of the dental provider community, she said.

Helgeson commented that the problem may have been defined incorrectly. It was defined as access to dental care, so a lot of energy was spent on thinking about how to get people into dental offices. He said that what is lacking is an effective oral health delivery system. The first step in exploring the development of such a system would be to determine where the majority of severe oral disease exists, which subpopulations are concentrated and where, and then think about how to reach those populations through collaborative efforts. Some of that work is underway, but more can be done to work from that health system core, and then build education and funding around that base, said Helgesen.

Online audience members noted the need to start reporting on the thousands of people currently experiencing mouth pain as a public health crisis. Focus on minimally invasive care and incentivizing what works is crucial, another said. Other thoughts included adding dental therapists to the equation, providing services in a transdisciplinary manner to meet unmet needs, and instilling the concept that oral health *is* overall health. For one virtual participant, including dental insurance as part of medical coverage to meet unmet needs was a critically important issue that has yet to be addressed.

The Needs of People with Disabilities

John Kemp brought up the mantra of the disability rights movement that stated: *nothing about us without us*, which has been more recently modified and improved to now simply state: *nothing without us*. This means there must be equity and equality for the participation of people with disabilities in all aspects of oral health promotion, disease prevention, and dental treatment. "We must do more," he insisted, and suggested one way forward would be to form a working group that looks at the holistic approach to policy reimbursement, care, and respect for the human dignity of all people. Kemp's remarks were embraced by one of the virtual participants who expressed support for creating continuing education groups and local communities to share information on how best to support people with disabilities. This would open opportunities for health professionals to learn from and with one another while partnering with persons with disabilities. Such communities of practice, suggested the participant, could meet regularly to discuss, test, and promote practice opportunities, continuity-of-care models, and the creation of dental homes within group homes and other community-based facilities or institutions.

Education

Paul Glassman shared his concern about some of the focus on education. There is an assumption that if education is changed, the care delivery will follow, which has not been supported by evidence. He mentioned that during his education, there was a rotation with medical students in conducting home visits. Despite the interprofessional exposure, most of his colleagues in the dental school never moved to that type of integrated care. This led him away from the belief that simply educating students differently will be enough to make a change. He said that it might be necessary to approach the idea of medical–dental integration from the other way around and start with changing delivery systems, which in turn can change education.

Daniel McNeil agreed with Glassman that education alone would not be enough to see downstream effects. However, he still sees a need for interprofessional education with dental students to prepare them for their careers as more holistic providers. He also wondered what the evidence is regarding the training of professionals, and how can that best be done to evoke change in the future? This is an action point for him coming out of this workshop, he said.

A dental student in the audience, John Button, thinks that interprofessional education and exposure to different career paths could start earlier. Discussing the different paths that careers can take while students are at the undergraduate level and still at a stage where they are willing to accept this information would be helpful. Further, he said that it is also important to consider the difficulties dental students face with the high cost of education. It is very challenging to graduate with high debts and then decide to work in a rural underserved community. Most recent graduates cannot afford to do that. There are some programs, but, he said, it would be helpful if the issue of financing education could be part of a national conversation on oral health for underserved communities.

CLOSING

In the final closing remarks, Kaz Rafia from the CareQuest Institute for Oral Health shared his thoughts that the participants understand the importance of collaboration and the immense value of learning from and leaning on each other for support. Stories of success and resilience were shared, and all have been confronted with the harsh realities of oral health inequities that persist. There was great conversation during the workshop, and the participants have come to appreciate the wealth of knowledge that each individual brings to the table, he said. The discussions revealed a frequently expressed vision of a world where every person has access to quality oral health care, independent of their level of ability or any other dynamic that might impede achieving optimal health care. He asked participants to carry forward the spirit of the workshop, to nurture the relationships formed, and build upon the knowledge gained. Together a global network of knowledge and exchange can be built where best practices are shared.

Appendix A

References

Akinlotan, M. A., and A. O. Ferdinand. 2020. Emergency department visits for nontraumatic dental conditions: A systematic literature review. *Journal of Public Health Dentistry* 80(4):313-326. https://doi.org/10.1111/jphd.12386.

American Academy of Pediatric Dentistry. 2023. Behavior guidance for the pediatric dental patient. In *Reference Manual of Pediatric Dentistry*. Chicago, IL: American Academy of Pediatric Dentistry. Pp. 359-377.

Bruen, B. K., E. Steinmetz, T. Bysshe, P. Glassman, and L. Ku. 2016. Potentially preventable dental care in operating rooms for children enrolled in Medicaid. *Journal of the American Dental Association* 147(9):702-708. https://doi.org/10.1016/j.adaj.2016.03.019.

CareQuest Institute for Oral Health. 2023. *Uninsured and in need: 68.5 million lack dental insurance, more may be coming.* https://www.carequest.org/resource-library/uninsured-and-need (accessed April 30, 2024).

Choi, B. C. K., and A. W. P. Pak. 2006. Multidisciplinarity, interdisciplinarity and trans-disciplinarity in health research, services, education and policy: 1. Definitions, objectives, and evidence of effectiveness. *Clinical & Investigative Medicine* 29(6):351-364.

CMS (Centers for Medicare & Medicaid Services). n.d.a. *Access to health coverage.* https://www.cms.gov/pillar/expand-access (accessed May 29, 2024).

CMS. n.d.b. *Value-based care.* https://www.cms.gov/priorities/innovation/key-concepts/value-based-care (accessed July 5, 2024).

CMS. 2023. *National health expenditure accounts.* https://www.cms.gov/data-research/statistics-trends-and-reports/national-health-expenditure-data/historical (accessed May 29, 2024).

CO-OP Chicago. n.d. *Coordinated oral health promotion (CO-OP) Chicago.* https://co-opchicago.ihrp.uic.edu/ (accessed May 29, 2024).

FDI (FDI World Dental Federation). n.d. *FDI's definition of oral health.* https://www.fdiworlddental.org/fdis-definition-oral-health (accessed July 5, 2024).

Glassman, P., A. Caputo, N. Dougherty, R. Lyons, Z. Messieha, C. Miller, B. Peltier, and M. Romer. 2009. Special care dentistry association consensus statement on sedation, anesthesia, and alternative techniques for people with special needs. *Special Care in Dentistry* 29(1):2-8. https://doi.org/10.1111/j.1754-4505.2008.00055.x.

Glick, M., D. M. Williams, D. V. Kleinman, M. Vujicic, R. G. Watt, and R. J. Weyant. 2016. A new definition for oral health developed by the FDI World Dental Federation opens the door to a universal definition of oral health. *Journal of the American Dental Association* 147(12):915-917. https://doi.org/10.1016/j.adaj.2016.10.001.

Heaton, L. J., M. Santoro, P. Martin, and E. P. Tranby. 2024. *Experiences with and outcomes of oral health care: Perspectives from nationally representative data.* Boston, MA: CareQuest Institute. https://doi.org/10.35565/CQI.2024.2001.

HHS (U.S. Department of Health and Human Services). 2000. *Oral health in America: A report of the surgeon general.* Rockville, MD: NIH National Institute of Dental and Craniofacial Research.

HRSA (Health Resources & Services Administration). 2024. *Health workforce shortage areas.* https://data.hrsa.gov/topics/health-workforce/shortage-areas (accessed July 5, 2024).

IPEC (Interprofessional Education Collaborative). 2023. *IPEC core competencies for interprofessional collaborative practice: Version 3.* Washington, DC: IPEC. https://www.ipecollaborative.org/assets/core-competencies/IPEC_Core_Competencies_Version_3_2023.pdf (accessed May 29, 2024).

John, M. T. 2022. Standardization of dental patient-reported outcomes measurement using OHIP-5—Validation of 'Recommendations for use and scoring of oral health impact profile versions.' *Journal of Evidence-Based Dental Practice* 22(1):101645. https://doi.org/10.1016/j.jebdp.2021.101645.

Lee, H. H., C. W. Lewis, B. Saltzman, and H. Starks. 2012. Visiting the emergency department for dental problems: Trends in utilization, 2001 to 2008. *American Journal of Public Health* 102(11):e77-e83. https://doi.org/10.2105/ajph.2012.300965.

Lee, H. H., C. W. Lewis, and C. M. McKinney. 2016. Disparities in emergency department pain treatment for toothache. *JDR Clinical & Translational Research* 1(3):226-233. https://doi.org/10.1177/2380084416655745.

Lee, H. H, C. W. Lehew, D. Avenetti, J. Buscemi, and A. Koerber. 2019. Understanding oral health behaviors among children treated for caries under general anesthesia. *Journal of Dentistry for Children* 86(2):101-108.

Lee, H. H., L. Faundez, C. Yarbrough, C. W. Lewis, and A. T. LoSasso. 2020a. Patterns in pediatric dental surgery under general anesthesia across 7 state Medicaid programs. *JDR Clinical & Translational Research* 5(4):358-365. https://doi.org/10.1177/2380084420906114.

Lee, H. H., L. Faundez, K. Nasseh, and A. T. LoSasso. 2020b. Does preventive care reduce severe pediatric dental caries? *Preventing Chronic Disease* 17. https://doi.org/10.5888/pcd17.200003.

Lee, H. H., L. Faundez, and A. T. LoSasso. 2020c. A cross-sectional analysis of community water fluoridation and prevalence of pediatric dental surgery among Medicaid enrollees. *JAMA Network Open* 3(8):e205882. https://doi.org/10.1001/jamanetworkopen.2020.5882.

Lewis, C. W., C. M. McKinney, H. H. Lee, M. L. Melbye, and T. C. Rue. 2015. Visits to US emergency departments by 20- to 29-year-olds with toothache during 2001-2010. *Journal of the American Dental Association* 146(5):295-302.e2. https://doi.org/10.1016/j.adaj.2015.01.013.

Lin, M., G. Thornton-Evans, S. O. Griffin, L. Wei, M. Junger, and L. Espinoza. 2018. Increased dental use may affect changes in treated and untreated dental caries in young children. *JDR Clinical & Translational Research* 4(1):49-57. https://doi.org/10.1177/2380084418793410.

Manski, R., F. Rohde, and T. Ricks. 2021. *Trends in the number and percentage of the population with any dental or medical visits, 2003-2018.* Statistical Brief 537. Rockville, MD: Agency for Healthcare Research and Quality. https://meps.ahrq.gov/data_files/publications/st537/stat537.shtml (accessed May 29, 2024).

Manski, R., F. Rohde, T. Ricks, and N. Chalmers. 2022. *Number and percentage of the population with any dental or medical visits by insurance coverage and geographic area, 2019.* Statistical Brief 544. Rockville, MD: Agency for Healthcare Research and Quality. https://meps.ahrq.gov/data_files/publications/st544/stat544.shtml (accessed May 29, 2024).

McNeil, D. W., C. L. Randall, S. Baker, B. Borrelli, J. M. Burgette, B. Gibson, L. J. Heaton, G. Kitsaras, C. McGrath, and J. T. Newton. 2022. Consensus statement on future directions for the behavioral and social sciences in oral health. *Journal of Dental Research* 101(6):619-622. https://doi.org/10.1177/00220345211068033.

NASEM (National Academies of Sciences, Engineering, and Medicine). 2023. *Achieving whole health: A new approach for veterans and the nation.* Washington, DC: The National Academies Press. https://doi.org/10.17226/26854.

NIH (National Institutes of Health). 2021. *Oral health in America: Advances and challenges.* Bethesda, MD: NIH National Institute of Dental and Craniofacial Research.

NIH. 2023. *NIH designates people with disabilities as a population with health disparities.* https://www.nih.gov/news-events/news-releases/nih-designates-people-with-disabilities-population-health-disparities (accessed July 5, 2024).

Pacific Center for Special Care. 2014. *The virtual dental home.* https://dental.pacific.edu/sites/default/files/users/user244/VirtualDentalHome_PolicyBrief_Aug_2014_HD_ForPrintOnly.pdf (accessed May 29, 2024).

PHOP (Prenatal Oral Health Program). n.d. *POHP.* https://www.prenataloralhealth.org/index.php/site/index (accessed June 4, 2024).

Sacramento County Department of Health. 2022. *Teeth for a lifetime? Oral health in Sacramento, 2022.* https://dhs.saccounty.gov/PUB/Documents/Oral%20Health/Sac%20County%20OH%20Needs%20Assessment%202022%20ADULT%20focus%20FINAL%20with%20clips.pdf (accessed May 29, 2024).

School-Based Health Alliance. 2023. *Findings from the 2022 National Census of School-Based Health Centers.* https://sbh4all.org/wp-content/uploads/2023/10/FINDINGS-FROM-THE-2022-NATIONAL-CENSUS-OF-SCHOOL-BASED-HEALTH-CENTERS-09.20.23.pdf (accessed May 29, 2024).

Stein Duker, L. I., D. H. Como, C. Jolette, C. Vigen, C. L. Gong, M. E. Williams, J. C. Polido, L. I. Flor{\'i}ndez-Cox, and S. A. Cermak. 2023. Sensory adaptations to improve physiological and behavioral distress during dental visits in autistic children. *JAMA Network Open* 6(6):e2316346. https://doi.org/10.1001/jamanetworkopen.2023.16346.

University of Illinois Chicago College of Dentistry. 2024. *PROTECT research study.* https://dentistry.uic.edu/protect-research-study/ (accessed May 29, 2024).

WHO (World Health Organization). 2024. *Oral health.* https://www.who.int/health-topics/oral-health#tab=tab_1 (accessed April 30, 2024).

Williams, W., E. Fisher, and N. Edwards. 2023a. *Bold action or slow decay? The state of NHS dentistry and future policy actions.* https://www.nuffieldtrust.org.uk/research/bold-action-or-slow-decay-the-state-of-nhs-dentistry-and-future-policy-actions (accessed April 30, 2024).

Williams, A.-R., A. Yaqub, P. Glassman, and V. Phillips. 2023b. Shortening-the-line: Reducing the need for sedation and general anesthesia for dental care for people with disabilities. *Journal of the California Dental Association* 51(1). https://doi.org/10.1080/19424396.2023.2253958.

Yarbrough, C., and M. Vujicic. 2019. Oral health trends for older Americans. *Journal of the American Dental Association* 150(8):714-716. https://doi.org/10.1016/j.adaj.2019.05.026.

Appendix B

Workshop Agenda

**EXPLORING HOLISTIC ORAL HEALTH VALUE
PROPOSITION FRAMEWORKS EMBEDDED WITHIN
A WHOLE HEALTH HOME: A WORKSHOP**

**GLOBAL FORUM ON INNOVATION IN
HEALTH PROFESSIONAL EDUCATION**

**Penn Dental Medicine
Corby Auditorium
240 S. 40th St
Philadelphia, PA 19104**

Workshop Objectives
- To understand the challenges faced by different interest groups in offering and receiving oral disease prevention and oral health promotion efforts.
- To learn from and with other professions and communities for a fuller understanding of each interest groups' pains and gains.
- To explore a value proposition for oral disease prevention, interprofessional oral health education, and payment models for demonstrating improved overall health of persons with mental and physical disabilities.

WORKSHOP AGENDA

Day 1: February 15, 2024

11:00–11:20 am ET	**Welcome** • Bruce Doll (Cochair), Office of Research, Uniformed Services University • Anita Duhl Glicken (Cochair), Executive Director, National Interprofessional Initiative on Oral Health
11:20–12:20 pm	**Session 1: Framing the Workshop Objectives** **Moderator:** Isabel Garcia, Dean, UF College of Dentistry, University of Florida **Panelists:** The value of oral health promotion and disease prevention to limit the need for costly/invasive interventions • Helen H. Lee, Associate Professor, Department of Anesthesiology, College of Medicine, University of Illinois Chicago and Director of Medical Scholars Program Oral disease prevention and oral health promotion to maximize oral health care experiences and outcomes for persons with disabilities • Paul Glassman, Associate Dean for Research and Community Engagement, College of Dental Medicine, California Northstate University Virtual Lifelong learning from and with other professions for oral disease prevention and oral health promotion • Karen Hall, Oral Health Integration Manager, Capitol Dental Care • Donna M. Hallas, Program Director, Pediatrics NP, New York University • Cynthia Lord, PA Clinician, Lake County Free Clinic • Teresa A. Marshall, Professor, University of Iowa • Daniel W. McNeil, College of Dentistry, University of Florida • Lemmietta McNeilly, Chief Staff Officer, American Speech-Language-Hearing Association **Audience Questions/Comments/Input**

12:20 pm	**Lunch in the Schattner Pavilion (40–45 minutes)**
1:00–2:15 pm	**Session 2: Understanding the Value Proposition**

Moderator: Robert J. Weyant, Professor and Chair, Department of Dental Public Health, University of Pittsburgh

What is a value proposition?

- Richard Berman, Associate Vice President for Strategic Initiatives for Innovation and Research, University of South Florida

Perspectives from different interest groups

Persons with disabilities

- John Kemp, President and CEO, Lakeshore Foundation

Providers/Educators (Interprofessional)

- Mark Deutchman, Associate Dean for Rural Health, University of Colorado, School of Medicine Virtual

Payers

- Randi Tillman, Executive Dental Director, Health Care Services Corporation Virtual

Policy Makers

- Natalia I. Chalmers Chief Dental Officer, Office of the Administrator, Centers for Medicare & Medicaid Services

Audience Questions/Comments/Input

2:15–3:10 pm   **Demonstrating the Value Proposition for Persons with Disabilities**

Question: What was the pain and gain for each or some of the interest groups discussed in the example?

Moderator and Opening Remarks: Mark Wolff, Dean, Penn Dental Medicine, University of Pennsylvania

Examples

- Leah I. Stein Duker, Assistant Professor, USC Chan Division of Occupational Science and Occupational Therapy Sensory Adapted Dental Environments for Children with Autism Spectrum Disorder: A Value Proposition Case Example—Virtual

- Betsy Lee White, Chief Operating Officer, Access Dental Care (a mobile Special Care Dentistry practice that serves people with disabilities and older adults in North Carolina)

3:10 pm   **Breakout Group Instructions**
- Bruce Doll (Cochair), Office of Research, Uniformed Services University
- Anita Duhl Glicken (Cochair), Executive Director, National Interprofessional Initiative on Oral Health

3:15–3:30 pm   **BREAK—15 minutes**

3:30–5:00 pm   **Three Breakout Groups:** Explore value proposition models for persons with disabilities. Each group is being assigned a lens through which it is asked to discuss a value proposition that demonstrates value to each interest group—persons with disabilities, interprofessional providers/educators, and payers/policy makers (max: 30/room)
NOTE: Attendees can choose to join a breakout group or stay in the main room
Breakout Groups: Exploring Value Propositions

Group 1. Value proposition through the lens of persons with disabilities (Room LL19A)
- Leads: Teresa A. Marshall and Daniel W. McNeil
- Staff: Sarah Flynn, Director, Strategic Development and Alumni Relations, Penn Dental Medicine

Group 2. Value proposition through the lens of IP providers/educators (Room LL20A)
- Leads: Jeffery Stewart and Cynthia Lord
- Staff: Julie Pavlin, Director, Board on Global Health, National Academies

Group 3. Value Proposition through the lens of the payers/policymakers (Room LL20B)
- Leads: Marko Vujicic & Donna M. Hallas
- Staff: Patricia Cuff, Director, Global Forum on Innovation in HPE, National Academies

3:30–5:00 pm   **Corby Auditorium/Main Room:** Explore interprofessional education and collaborative practice for holistic oral health promotion and prevention for underserved communities.
Session 3: Whole Health Through Oral Health Examples
- **Moderator:** Robert J. Weyant, Professor and Chair, Department of Dental Public Health, University of Pittsburgh
- **Staff:** Erika Chow, Research Assistant, Global Forum on Innovation in HPE, National Academies

Central Health and Wellness Center: Providing Holistic Health for Children and the Local Community (a holistic approach to oral health through school-based health centers)
- Karen Hall, Oral Health Integration Manager, Capitol Dental Care

Oral Health for Mental Health Patients Project in Zimbabwe (SUD clinic with oral disease prevention services and interprofessional learning)
- Cleopatra Matanhire, Director, Oral Ling Axis Trust; and Department of Oral Health, University of Zimbabwe
- Kudzai Murembwe-Machingauta, Training coordinator, Oral Ling Axis Trust; and Technical Lead Covid Go at OPHID, Africa University, Zimbabwe

Oral Health into General Health: A Mother-Child-Vaccination Program to reduce Early Childhood Caries in Peru
- Rita S. Villena, Chair of the Pediatric Dentistry Department, University San Martin de Porres, Peru

Putting Families First (a University of Florida interprofessional course that make regular in-person home visits to the volunteer families' homes to help determine ways for the families to maintain or improve their health) Virtual
- Olga S. Ensz, Director of Community-Based Outreach, University of Florida

Mini Mouth Care Matters: Empowering medical and allied health care professionals to make every contact count
- Urshla Devalia, Consultant Pediatric Dentist, Eastman Dental Hospital, UCLH (London); National Lead for Mini Mouth Care Matters

5:00 pm   **Adjourn to Reception in Schattner Pavilion,**
                   Courtesy of Penn Dental Medicine, light hors d'oeuvres served
                   Optional tour of Penn Dental Medicine Care Center for Persons with Disabilities

5:00–6:00 pm   **Workshop Planning Committee subgroup:** Go to room (LL20A) to debrief and plan for Day 2.

6:30 pm   Workshop Planning Committee:
                   Dinner at the hotel* People with physical, sensory, intellectual, mental health, and non-apparent disabilities

Day 2: February 16, 2024

8:00 am ET   **Breakfast in Schattner Pavilion**

9:00–9:05 am   **Welcome Back**
                   - Bruce Doll (Cochair), Office of Research, Uniformed Services University
                   - Anita Duhl Glicken (Cochair), Executive Director, National Interprofessional Initiative on Oral Health

9:05–9:30 am   **Breakout Group Presentation of Draft Value Proposition**
                   - Planning Committee
                   Questions for the audience

                   Session 4: Fitting the Value Proposition into the Larger Picture
                   - **Moderator:** Teresa A. Marshall, Professor, University of Iowa

9:30–10:00 am	**Presentation on Equity** • Michael Helgeson, Chief Executive Officer, Apple Tree Dental Discussion with participants
10:00–10:30 am	**Whole Health Home** Learning from and with other professions in a "holistic oral health home" that could be in a dental office, medical clinic, school, home, church, pharmacy, etc. • Michael Glick, Executive Director of the Center for Integrative Global Oral Health and Professor of Clinical Restorative Dentistry at Penn Dental Medicine Discussion with participants
10:30–10:45 am	**BREAK—15 minutes**
10:45–11:00 am	**Session 5: Closing** **A Value Proposition Revisited** • Planning Committee Participant input
11:00–11:45 am	**Roundtable open discussion** **Facilitator:** Bruce Doll (Cochair), Office of Research, Uniformed Services University • Workshop planning committee offers reflections • Participants and speakers offer additional comments
11:45–12:00 pm	**Closing remarks** • Kaz Rafia, Chief Health Equity Officer, Executive Vice President, CareQuest Institute for Oral Health • Bruce Doll (Cochair), Office of Research, Uniformed Services University
12:00 pm	**Adjourn**
12:00–1:00 pm	**Workshop Planning Committee:** Optional debrief lunch (Room LL20A)

Appendix C

Workshop Planning Committee Biographical Sketches

Anita Glicken, M.S.W. (*Cochair*), is associate dean and professor emeritus at the University of Colorado Anschutz Medical Center and has over 35 years of administrative, research, and education experience. She was a founding member, and now serves as the executive director, of the National Interprofessional Initiative on Oral Health (NIIOH) and is an active member of the Santa Fe group. Glicken is immediate past chair of Health Resources and Services Administration's Advisory Committee on Training in Primary Care Medicine and Dentistry and past chair of the Primary Care Collaborative's Advisory Committee for the Integration of Oral Health in Primary Care Compendium project. Glicken has personally received several national awards; under her leadership, the NIIOH has received the ADEA Gies Foundation's Gies Award and the National Center for Interprofessional Practice and Education's George T. Thibault Award. She has been a consultant to the National Academies of Medicine Oral Health Integration Workshop and currently serves on the Advisory Group for the Centers for Disease Control and Prevention–funded National Association of Chronic Disease Directors' Medical–Dental Integration Project and the Meharry University Oral Health Equity Project.

Glicken has served on several national expert panels to develop tools and resources supporting workforce research, practice, and policy, including HRSA's National Center for Health Workforce Analysis (NCHWA) on Data and Methods for Tracking, Supply, Demand, Distribution, and Adequacy of the Primary Care Workforce; HRSA's 2014 report, *Integration of Oral Health and Primary Care Practice*; and the Qualis Health White Paper, *Oral Health: An Essential Component of Primary Care*. Past leadership roles include president of the Physician Assistant Education Association and President/CEO of the National Commission on Certification of Physician Assistants Health Foundation, where she worked with HRSA's National Center for Health Workforce Analysis to create a database on certified physician assistant practice to inform health policy and workforce planning.

A clinical social worker, Glicken's career has focused on health care transformation, partnering to create innovative education and care delivery models grounded in interprofessional collaboration and health equity. She was project director of an American International Health Alliance PEPFAR contract to create new educational programs to build indigenous mid-level health workforce capacity in South Africa. Glicken is the author of more than 100 publications in health care education, workforce, and research.

Bruce Doll, D.D.S., Ph.D., M.B.A. (*Cochair*), is the assistant vice president for technological research and innovation, Office of Research at Uniformed Services University (USU) in Bethesda, Maryland. He leads the development and integration of database management within the research portfolio and the advancement of novel technologies focused upon military medical requirements. His formal education includes a D.D.S. from SUNY Buffalo, periodontics specialty certificate from Navy Postgraduate Dental School, Ph.D. from Penn State, and an M.B.A. from the Navy Postgraduate School. During 34 years of service with the U.S. Navy, he served with both the Navy and U.S. Marine Corps, INCONUS and OCONUS. Several times deployed, RADM Doll completed his service as both director, Research, Development and Acquisition Directorate for the Defense Health Agency in Falls Church, Virginia, and the Deputy Commander, U.S. Army Medical Research and Materiel Command, Fort Detrick, Maryland, overseeing execution of medical research funded by the Defense Health Program. He has had academic appointments with Carnegie Mellon University, University of Pittsburgh, Oregon Health Sciences University, University of Maryland, Pennsylvania State University, and Rutgers University prior to coming to USU. He served as the chief operating officer for the Rutgers–Cleveland Clinic Consortium for the Armed Forces Institute of Regenerative Medicine. He has served on several scientific boards. He has published on the topics of bone regeneration and is a former grantee of the National Institutes of Health and the National Institute of Standards and Technology.

Richard Berman, M.B.A., M.P.H., is the associate vice president for strategic initiatives for innovation and research at the University of South Florida, visiting social entrepreneurship professor in the Muma College of Business, and a professor in the Institute for Advanced Discovery & Innovation. He is currently an elected member of the National Academy of Medicine (formerly known as the Institute of Medicine) of the National Academy of

Sciences in Washington, D.C., and is a board member for Emblem Health. He is a member of the Seeds of Peace Board of Directors, a board member for the Savannah Centre for Diplomacy, Democracy and Development in Abuja, Nigeria, and CATAYS, Inc. Additionally, he is the vice-chair of the board of directors for OIC of South Florida. Previous organizations in which he has served on the board of directors include the Lillian Vernon Corporation, the Westchester Jewish Chronicle (chairman of the advisory board), the American Jewish Committee (Westchester Chapter), and the March of Dimes. Previously, Berman has worked as a management consultant for McKinsey & Company, the executive vice president of NYU Medical Center, and professor of health care management at the NYU School of Medicine. He served as the special advisor to the leader of the African Union-United Nations Peace Keeping Mission in Darfur. He has also held various roles at Korn Ferry International, Howe-Lewis International, served in two cabinet positions in New York State government, and the U.S. Department of Health, Education, and Welfare. In 1995, Berman was selected by Manhattanville College to serve as its 10th President. Berman received his B.B.A., M.B.A., and M.P.H. from the University of Michigan and holds honorary doctorates from Manhattanville College and New York Medical College.

Urshla (Oosh) Devalia, B.D.S., is a pediatric dental consultant working at the Eastman Dental Hospital, University College Hospital, London and in the Community Dental Services (CDS) in Bedfordshire. She is also the Managed Clinical Network chair for pediatric dentistry in the East of England. Devalia is also the national lead for Mini Mouth Care Matters (Mini MCM), an initiative created to empower medical and allied health care professionals to make every contact count by educating on the importance of integrating mouth care with general health. She is also lead for the pilot project scheme run by the Eastman Dental Education Centre & Health Education England titled Child Focused Dental Practices, which is a national scheme being delivered in primary care dental practices across three National Health Service regions (the South West, London, and the East of England). A trustee and board member of the Executive Committee for the British Society of Pediatric Dentistry, she contributes to a number of briefing papers to improve health and social care for children and young people across the UK with her primary focus on the management of vulnerable patient groups, including those with learning disabilities and/or autism, and those with complex medical needs. She worked for a number of years as clinical policy lead for the Office of the Chief Dental Officer for England, looking to ensure barriers and inequalities are removed for children and young people with additional needs who attend special education settings. A member of the Institute of Leadership and Management, she believes in cross-sectional working, ensuring gaps in workforce are addressed across England.

Karen Hall, R.D.H., E.P.D.H., graduated in 1985 from Oregon Health Sciences University with a degree in dental hygiene. Currently serving as oral health integration manager for Capitol Dental Care, she creates opportunities for a fantastic team of oral health providers to provide dental services for underserved community members in nontraditional settings. Focusing on public and community health since 1999, she has implemented new models of dental delivery that increase quality dental access and engage new partnerships for integrative efforts. Hall spent several years working alongside medical and mental health providers in school-based health centers; created oral health education series for medical, dental, traditional health worker, childcare, and senior care providers; and has sat on numerous committees within the coordinated care organizations who manage Medicaid benefits for Oregonians. In 2018, Hall was the second dental hygienist in the state to be awarded the Oregon Dental Hygienists' Association Access to Care Award, and she currently sits on the board of the Oregon Dental Hygienists' Association as advocacy director.

Donna Hallas, Ph.D., PPCNP-BC, CPNP, PMHS, FAANP, FAAN, is a clinical professor and director of the Pediatric Nurse Practitioner Program at New York University Meyers College of Nursing. She maintains a practice as a pediatric nurse practitioner in primary care with a focus on developmental and behavioral health. She has presented at national and international conferences on implementation of evidence-based practice in ambulatory pediatric health care centers. She has presented on all aspects of oral health assessment and care management for pediatric and adolescent patients. She has conducted research on educating mothers about oral health needs during the postpartum period to prevent cavities in young children. She works collaboratively with dental faculty to improve the oral health care of children from diverse populations. She is published in peer-reviewed journals on the oral health care needs of young children. Her most recent research has been on vaccine hesitancy in which she conducted and published a quasi-experimental intervention study to vaccinate pregnant people and infants within the first 6 months of life. She is the editor in chief for the *Journal of Pediatric Health Care.*

John D. Kemp, Esq., is president and CEO of Lakeshore Foundation, which is an internationally recognized organization providing opportunities for individuals with physical disability and chronic health conditions to lead healthy, active, independent lives. Located in Birmingham, Alabama, Lakeshore also serves as a U.S. Olympic and Paralympic

Training site, a center for research and with the disability community, a strong advocate for inclusion. Kemp launched his most recent and widely acclaimed book, *Disability Friendly: How to Move from Clueless to Inclusive* (Wiley, 2022). Widely respected for his many achievements in the corporate and nonprofit worlds and his leadership in the disability movement, Kemp, a person with a disability, cofounded the American Association of People with Disabilities and has held a variety of CEO and senior executive positions with national and international nonprofits. He was honored with the Henry B. Betts Award, widely regarded as America's highest honor for disability leadership and service. He is also the recipient of the Dole Leadership Prize, joining a prestigious group of international recipients including Nelson Mandela and two former U.S. Presidents. In addition, Kemp serves on Delta Air Lines' Advisory Board on Disability. A graduate of Georgetown University and Washburn University School of Law, Kemp and his wife, Sameta, enjoy spending time with their family, including five grandsons.

Cynthia Lord, M.H.S., PA-C, earned her PA from Yale University, and has spent much of her 32-year career working in primary care and academia. Currently, she works as a PA at Lake County Free Clinic in Painesville, Ohio. A PA educator for 29 years, she has spent most of her time as a PA program director, most recently as founder of the Case Western Reserve University PA program and cofounder of the Quinnipiac University PA program. She has served on numerous oral health advisory boards including the National Interprofessional Initiative on Oral Health, the national PA Oral Health Advisory Group, the Connecticut Oral Health Initiative, and as a contributor to the 2014 HRSA Oral Health Competencies. She currently serves on the board of Oral Health Ohio and is the Ohio oral health champion for the Center for Integration of Primary Care and Oral Health, helping Ohio health professions programs integrate oral health into their curriculum. A contributor on a Case Western Reserve School of Dental Medicine National Institute of Dental and Craniofacial Research grant, she was a member of an interprofessional team working to improve access to dental care for low-income children in Cleveland. Her scholarship includes numerous presentations, abstracts, and poster presentations around oral health and interprofessional education.

Cleopatra Matanhire-Zihanzu, B.D.S., M.B.A., M.Sc., is the director of the Oral Lung Axis Trust, and a faculty member in the Department of Oral Health, Faculty of Medicine and Health Sciences, University of Zimbabwe. She is an oral health advocate who applies translational research for dental education advancement and oral health policy development. Matanhire-Zihanzu is a cofounding member of the Oral Health for Mental Health

Patients Project Zimbabwe, currently in its third year of running. The project goal is transformation of oral health care of mental health patients in Zimbabwe to international best practice, through research, health education material development, and information dissemination. Matanhire-Zihanzu's responsibilities included project planning and management, grant applications, report writing, and coordinating interdisciplinary collaboration of oral and mental health interest groups in and out of Zimbabwe.

The project has seen Matanhire-Zihanzu awarded the 2021 Zimbabwe Dental Association Protea Award for the most contribution to the dental profession, 2022 Zimbabwe Dental Association Research Award, and the Zimbabwe Dental Association Research Award 2023. The project team to date has been awarded the International Dental Federation (FDI) World Dental Development Fund Grant Award for Oral Health Care for Mental Health Patients Project, Zimbabwe 2020; Zimbabwe Dental Association Presidential Award for notable outstanding dentistry project 2022; and the Partnership for Education Training and Research Advancement Mentorship Research Scholars Award 2023 courtesy of the University of Zimbabwe in collaboration with Stanford University and University of Denver Colorado, among other academic institutions. Matanhire-Zihanzu holds a bachelor of dental surgery, a master's in business administration, and a master of science in global health. She is also a 2017 Mandela Washington Fellow in Civic Leadership (Kansas State University) and a 2020–2021 Beit-Glasgow Scholar (University of Glasgow).

Teresa A. Marshall, Ph.D., is a registered dietitian and professor in the Department of Preventive and Community Dentistry, the Michael W. Finkelstein Centennial Professor of Teaching, and the director of the Student Research Program at the University of Iowa's College of Dentistry. Her primary research interests focus on the relationships among diet, nutrition, oral health, and systemic health. Marshall has engaged with national and international groups to understand, educate, and advocate for caries prevention with emphasis on diet. Her efforts in oral health–nutrition education were recognized by the American Society of Nutrition, which awarded her the 2020 Roland L. Weinsier Award for Excellence in Medical/ Dental Nutrition Education. She is a member of the Academy of Nutrition and Dietetics (including the practice group Nutrition Educators of Health Professionals), American Dental Association, International Association for Dental Research, American Dental Education Association, American Society for Nutrition, and a board member of the American Academy of Cariology. She is a research editor for the *Journal of the Academy of Nutrition and Dietetics*. She completed a dietetic internship and a doctorate in human nutrition at the University of Iowa.

Daniel W. McNeil, Ph.D., is an endowed professor and chair of the Department of Community Dentistry and Behavioral Science at the University of Florida College of Dentistry. He also serves as director of the Southeast Center for Research to Reduce Disparities in Oral Health. He has a Ph.D. in clinical psychology from the University of Alabama, and a postdoctoral fellowship in clinical health psychology and behavioral dentistry at the University of Florida. McNeil is a researcher in health psychology, including behavioral dentistry, studying anxiety, pain, and their interaction, with a focus on dental anxiety, fear, and phobia. McNeil has had sabbaticals at the University of Sydney and was a Fulbright Senior Fellow in New Zealand. In 2021, he received the Distinguished Scientist Award for Behavioral, Epidemiologic, and Health Services Research from the International Association for Dental Research. As a lead organizer of the 2020 international conference "Behavioral and Social Oral Health Sciences Summit," this initiative resulted in his being a first author on a "Consensus Statement" publication in the *Journal of Dental Research*. Additionally, he was a lead editor for a 2023 special issue of *Community Dentistry and Oral Epidemiology* that provided a proceedings and extension from the Summit.

Lemmietta McNeilly, Ph.D., CCC-SLP, CAE, FASAE, FNAP, serves as the American Speech-Language-Hearing Association's (ASHA's) chief staff officer, speech-language pathology, and is responsible for the following units: Government Affairs and Public Policy, Speech-Language Pathology Practices (Clinical Issues, Health Care, and School Services), Special Interest Group Program, and International Programs. McNeilly is a distinguished scholar and fellow of the National Academies of Practice (NAP) as well as a member of the NAP Diversity, Equity, and Inclusion Task Force. She serves on the International Association of Communication Sciences and Disorders Board of Directors. She is an American Speech-Language-Hearing Association fellow, a fellow of the American Society of Association Executives (ASAE), a Certified Association Executive, and a Diversity Executive Leadership Scholar. She currently serves on the ASAE Board of Directors and ASAE Foundation Board. She consults with the World Health Organization and serves on the World Rehabilitation Alliance as a member of the Workforce Workstream. Previous appointments include serving as founding chair of the Department of Communication Sciences and Disorders at Florida International University, faculty at the University of Florida and Howard University, chair of the ASAE International Section Council and Healthcare Committee, National Coalition of Health Care Professionals Executive Board Secretary/Treasurer, and Executive Committee member. McNeilly has research experience and clinical expertise in developmental language disorders and dysphagia for medically fragile pediatrics. She is known internationally and has published and conducted seminars for leaders in health care associations and academic arenas on several topics including genomics for health care professionals, educating health professionals regarding social determinants of health, the International Classification of Health Functioning and Disability, practicing at the top of the license, interprofessional education and collaborative practice, speech-language pathology assistants, competency-based education, and assessing and managing the needs of culturally and linguistically diverse children with chronic health conditions.

Kudzai Murembwe-Machingauta, M.B.Ch.B., M.S., M.P.H., is a distinguished medical professional, currently serving as the technical lead for the integration of Covid-19 and mental health into HIV care and treatment for the Organization of Public Health Interventions and Development. She was previously curative services manager and acting director health services for Mutare City Council from 2018 to 2021. Machingauta's expertise lies in public health, backed by a master of public health degree from Africa University, a master of science in respiratory medicine from the University of South Wales, and bachelor of medicine and bachelor of surgery degrees from the University of Zimbabwe. She also holds certificates in project management and leadership and management in global health from the University of Washington and is an Implementation Science Fellow with PETRA (Basic Oral Health Package of Care for Mental Health Patients).

Her passion for public health has led her to implement numerous public health programs and actively participate in capacity building among health care workers in Zimbabwe. She is also a visionary of the Oral Lung Axis Trust, an association aimed at improving oral and lung health care worldwide. Machingauta's exceptional contributions have been recognized with the Cimas Prize and Dr. Dodge book prize for being the best M.P.H. student in the class of 2022. She is also an alumnus of the Merck Foundation Scholarship and the Joshua Nkomo Scholarship funds.

Jeffery Stewart, D.D.S., M.S., is currently a consultant at the American Dental Education Association (ADEA) where he formerly served as senior vice president for interprofessional and global collaboration. Prior to joining ADEA, he had been a faculty member at three dental schools where he was active in interprofessional education initiatives. He currently represents ADEA as a member of the Interprofessional Education Collaborative Planning Committee/Advisory Group and the Interprofessional Professionalism Collaborative. He attended college at the University of Delaware and received his dental degree from the University of North Carolina. Following a hospital general practice residency, he attended the University of Michigan, earning a master's degree in oral pathology and diagnosis.

Rita Villena, D.D.S., Ph.D., graduated from the Peruvian University Cayetano Heredia in Lima, Peru, with her master's and Ph.D. studies in pediatric dentistry at the Sao Paulo University–Brazil. She has been chair of the Pediatric Dentistry Department at San Martin de Porres University in Lima, Peru, since 2010. She is a member of the technical group of the Peruvian Ministry of Health and a member of the Vision 2030 Implementation and Monitoring working group of the FDI. She was the winner of the research Hatton Award for the Brazilian Division–International Association for Dental Research (IADR) (1997) and has held several positions at IADR including past president of the Peruvian Division–IADR (2003–2005) and past president and board member of the Latin American Region of the IADR (2011–2014), past president of the Peruvian Association of Dentistry for Infants (2012–2016) and chair of the Regional Development Program–IADR (2012–2014).

Villena has been conducting research in the field of prevention and pediatric dentistry for the past 20 years, with special interest in infancy. She is a clinician working together with pediatricians in private practice since 2000 and is the general co-coordinator of the Dental Caries Research Observatory for Children and Adolescents of the Latin American Region–IADR. She is an international speaker and has authored 14 book chapters in the Latin American region and publications in indexed journals. She is also part of the editorial boards of several international journals.

Marko Vujicic, Ph.D., currently serves as chief economist and vice president of the Health Policy Institute at the American Dental Association. He is a recognized thought leader in health care policy as it relates to dental care. He has published extensively in peer-reviewed journals such as *Health Affairs* and the *New England Journal of Medicine*, and his team's work is regularly cited by *CNN*, the *New York Times*, the *Wall Street Journal*, *Fox News*, and other media outlets. Previously, he was senior economist with the World Bank in Washington, D.C., where he focused on health systems reform in developing countries.

Vujicic holds several academic appointments. He is adjunct senior fellow at the Leonard Davis Institute of Health Economics, University of Pennsylvania, and affiliate faculty at the Center for Health and the Social Sciences, University of Chicago, as well as the Center for Health Services and Policy Research at the University of British Columbia. He is an adjunct professor at the University of Toronto and a visiting assistant professor at Tufts University.

Vujicic obtained his Ph.D. in economics from the University of British Columbia and a bachelor's degree in business from McGill University in Montreal.

Robert Weyant, M.S., D.M.D., Dr.P.H., is professor and chair of the Department of Dental Public Health, professor of epidemiology, and on the faculty of the Clinical and Translational Sciences Institute at the University of Pittsburgh. Weyant's research involves epidemiological research related to oral health disparities, the social determinants of health, and oral disease etiology. His research includes studies of gene-by-environment interactions, the linkages between oral and general health, and strategies for improving medical and dental integration.

Weyant has participated on three prior National Academies' committees: Temporomandibular Disorders: Priorities for Research and Care, Committee on Implementing High-Quality Primary Care, and Advancing Oral Health in America, and participated in the National Academies' workshop Sharing and Exchanging Ideas and Experiences on Community-Engaged Approaches to Oral Health. Weyant is a commissioner on the Lancet Commission on Global Oral Health where he is working on policy development for improving oral health care delivery. He is a diplomate of the American Board of Dental Public Health and is the editor in chief of the *Journal of Public Health Dentistry*. He was the recipient of the American Association for Dental Research/American Dental Association Evidence-Based Dentistry Faculty Award. He is recognized with this award for his lifelong contributions to evidence-based dentistry. He received his M.P.H. and dental degree from the University of Pittsburgh and a doctorate in epidemiology from the University of Michigan.

Mark S. Wolff, D.D.S., Ph.D., is the Morton Amsterdam Dean of the University of Pennsylvania School of Dental Medicine and a professor in the Department of Preventative and Restorative Dentistry. He has designed, developed, and implemented an extensive curriculum in caries risk assessment and has designed dental information systems to assist dental schools in monitoring the risk of the entire dental patient population.

Wolff started his dental career as a private practitioner, creating a family practice that focused on medically compromised and disabled patients of all ages. He has been a lifelong advocate and educator for individuals with physical, intellectual, and developmental disabilities through the lifespan. Wolff received his D.D.S. degree and Ph.D. in oral biology and pathology from Stony Brook University. He has served as the principal or coprincipal investigator on multiple benchtop and clinical research projects investigating dental caries, novel remineralizing agents, dental erosion, periodontal disease, dental materials, and dentinal hypersensitivity. He has coauthored more than 100 scientific papers and text chapters, and edited multiple textbooks. Wolff lectures worldwide and is a frequent consultant to industry. He served as associate dean at Stony Brook University School of Dental Medicine, where he helped develop and implement the first completely computerized dental record. Under his leadership, Penn Dental Medicine implemented extensive clinical programs of caries and health risk assessments, minimal intervention dentistry, tobacco cessation, evidence-based dental education, community-based dentistry, and dental care for all patients through the life course.

PLANNING COMMITTEE CONSULTANTS

Julian Fisher, B.D.S., M.Sc., M.I.H., is a policy advisor and analyst specializing in health workforce education, social and environmental determinants of health, and global oral health. He is currently based in Germany with regular monthly trips to UN agencies in Switzerland. He is also director, Advocacy and Networks, in a part-time capacity for the nongovernmental organization THEnet Training for Health Equity (New York). As chair of two World Health Organization (WHO) technical advisory groups, he is engaged in supporting WHO's technical and normative work.

Fisher was previously associate director, professional and scientific affairs, with the World Dental Federation, Geneva, Switzerland. His experience covers a diverse range of professional domains including international public health policy and advocacy (consultancies for WHO, UNESCO, and United National Environment Programme), health profession (federation) management, and health workforce undergraduate and postgraduate education. His work has been based in Europe, Tanzania, South Africa, Saudi Arabia, Falkland Islands, and Antarctica within various sectors and organizations. Julian Fisher earned his B.D.S. (dentistry) from Birmingham University in 1985, his M.Sc. (HIV/AIDS) from Stellenbosch University in 2002, and his M.I.H. (international health) from Charité University in 2006.

Isabel Garcia, D.D.S., M.P.H., joined the University of Florida College of Dentistry as dean on February 16, 2015, after retiring from the U.S. Public Health Service (USPHS) in 2014 as a rear admiral lower half. Garcia's career spans over 40 years in public health, clinical practice, research, teaching, and administration at the local, state, and national levels. Garcia joined the National Institute of Dental and Craniofacial Research (NIDCR) at the NIH in 1995 and held multiple leadership roles during her time there. She led NIDCR's science transfer efforts, directed the Institute's Office of Science Policy and Analysis, and served as acting NIDCR director from 2010 to 2011. Garcia also served as the institute's coordinator for global health and directed NIDCR's Residency in Dental Public Health program from 2005 to 2014. While with the USPHS, Garcia was deployed to help prepare a major health diplomacy mission to Central and South America, which provided care to over 85,000 people in 12 countries.

As deputy director of NIDCR from 2007 to 2014, she shared responsibility for the oversight and management of programs and functions within the institute, which included over 400 scientists and administrators dedicated to research, training, science policy, health education, communications, and financial management. Garcia received a doctorate in dental surgery from Virginia Commonwealth University and a master's degree in public health from the University of Michigan. She subsequently completed a residency in dental public health at the University of Michigan and a fellowship in primary care policy from the U.S. Public Health Service. A fellow of the American College of Dentists and the Pierre Fauchard Academy, Garcia is a diplomate and Past President of the American Board of Dental Public Health and an active member of the American Dental Education Association, the International Association for Dental Research, and the American Dental Association.

Michael Glick, D.M.D., is executive director of the Center for Integrative Global Oral Health and Fields-Rayant Professor at Penn Dental Medicine. From 2009 to 2015, Glick served as dean of the University at Buffalo, SUNY, School of Dental Medicine, where he remained as professor of oral diagnostic sciences before coming to Penn Dental Medicine in 2021. Prior to Buffalo, he was professor of oral medicine at Arizona School of Dentistry and Oral Health, A.T. Still University, also holding the post of associate dean of oral-medical sciences at the University's School of Osteopathic Medicine. While at the University of Medicine and Dentistry of New Jersey from 2001 to 2007, Glick served as chairman of the Department of Diagnostic Sciences and as director of both the Division of Oral Medicine and the Postgraduate Training Program in Oral Medicine. This position with Penn Dental Medicine is Glick's second faculty appointment, previously serving from 1994 to 2001 on the oral medicine faculty. During that time, he also directed the school's programs for medically complex patients and infectious diseases.

A widely published and respected lecturer, Glick served as editor in chief of *Journal of the American Dental Association* from 2005 to 2020. Globally, Glick has been active with the FDI World Dental Federation since 2007, serving on multiple committees including cochairing the Task Team Vision 2030. He also had a leading role in establishing FDI's Vision 2020 and most recently was the primary author of its Vision 2030, giving guidance for a global interdisciplinary and integrative role for oral health.

Zohray M. Talib, M.D. (*Forum Cochair*), is Executive Vice Dean, senior associate dean of academic affairs, chair of the Department of Medical Education and professor of medical education and medicine at the California University of Science and Medicine. Her experience spans the field of medical education and global health, with a focus on social accountability in health professions education. She has worked with undergraduate and graduate medical education programs in the United States and across sub-Saharan Africa to bring best practices into medical education, especially in low-resource settings. Talib's interests include community-based education, decentralized training, and building a robust and diverse faculty workforce for underserved communities. Talib led a study across 10 countries in Africa that shed light on the value of bringing learners into community-based health care settings. She also partnered with faculty in Africa to examine the burden of mental health and strategies to integrate mental health into primary care. Talib holds visiting faculty appointments at the Aga Khan University in East Africa as well as Mbarara University of Science and Technology in Uganda.

Talib brings to the field of academic medicine and global health the unique perspective of being a primary care physician, educator, and researcher. She teaches clinical medicine, health policy, and health systems to undergraduate medical students. Talib holds an adjunct faculty appointment at the George Washington University where she was previously associate program director for the internal medicine program and a researcher with the Health Workforce Institute.

Appendix D

Workshop Speaker
Biographical Sketches

Natalia Chalmers, D.D.S., M.H.Sc., Ph.D., is a board-certified pediatric dentist, oral health policy expert, and public health advocate who brings more than 20 years of clinical, research, industry, and regulatory experience to the Centers for Medicare & Medicaid Services (CMS) in her role as chief dental officer in the Office of the Administrator. Previously, Chalmers served as a dental officer at the U.S. Food and Drug Administration. She has devoted her career to transforming scientific and health care data and information into actionable insights to address equity, improve care, and better inform policy and funding. Chalmers completed her doctor of dental surgery degree at the Faculty of Dental Medicine of the Medical University of Sofia, a residency in pediatric dentistry at the University of Maryland School of Dentistry, a Ph.D. in oral microbiology from the Graduate Partnerships Program of the University of Maryland School of Dentistry and the National Institute for Dental and Craniofacial Research (NIDCR) at the National Institutes of Health (NIH), postdoctoral fellowship at the Forsyth Institute, and clinical research fellowship at NIDCR/NIDCR.

Chalmers holds a master's degree in clinical research from Duke Medical University and a certificate in drug development and regulatory science from the University of California San Francisco School of Pharmacy. Her research has translated into action, improving oral care and advocating for the role health policy can play across the lifespan—particularly when it embraces dental well-being as a facet of care for the whole person.

Mark Deutchman, M.D., is a professor in the Department of Family Medicine at the University of Colorado School of Medicine, School of

Dental Medicine and School of Public Health. He is associate dean for rural health at the University of Colorado and has served as director of the Colorado Area Health Education Centers system. He practiced family medicine in rural Washington State for 12 years. Since leaving rural practice he has been developing programs, conducting research, and teaching medical students, residents, and fellows with an emphasis on preparation for rural practice, maternity care, interprofessional collaboration, and oral health integration. He has served as an author for the *Smiles for Life* national oral health curriculum, helped found the Cavity Free at Three program in Colorado, and worked with the Medical Oral Expanded Care program. He completed medical school at the Ohio State University and family medicine residency in Spokane, Washington.

Olga S. Ensz, D.M.D., M.P.H., is a clinical assistant professor and director of community-based outreach with the University of Florida College of Dentistry (UFCD) Department of Community Dentistry and Behavioral Science. Ensz is a Florida native and a triple-gator, graduating from the University of Florida with her B.S. in nutrition in 2011, her D.M.D. degree in 2015, and a master of public health degree in 2018. She is currently pursuing a part-time residency in dental public health at the Boston University Henry M. Goldman School of Dental Medicine. Ensz has a strong passion for dental public health, interprofessional education, and oral health promotion and disease prevention in vulnerable populations. She currently oversees the department's school- and community-based dental outreach programs in Alachua and Collier counties and supervises dental students as they provide preventive dental services for pediatric patients at high risk for oral health problems. Ensz is the chief UFCD representative on the UF Health Sciences Center Interprofessional Education Committee, and currently serves as an Area Health Education Centers program liaison for the college.

Paul Glassman, D.D.S., M.A., M.B.A., is the associate dean for research and community engagement at the College of Dental Medicine at California Northstate University in Elk Grove, California, and professor emeritus at the University of the Pacific, Arthur A. Dugoni School of Dentistry in San Francisco. He has served on many national panels including the Institute of Medicine's (IOM) Committee on Oral Health Access to Services, which produced the IOM report *Improving Access to Oral Health Care for Vulnerable and Underserved Populations.*

Glassman has had many years of dental practice experience treating patients with complex conditions and has published and lectured extensively in the areas of hospital dentistry, dentistry for patients with special needs, dentistry for individuals with medical disabilities, dentistry for patients with dental fear, geriatric dentistry, and oral health systems reform. He has a long career working with special populations in a variety of practice and community settings. Glassman has been principal investigator (PI) or co-PI on over $32 million in grants and contracts over the last 30 years, focused on community-service demonstration and research programs designed to improve oral health for people with disabilities and other underserved populations. Glassman is a pioneer and has led the national movement to improve oral health using telehealth-connected teams and Virtual Dental Homes. Glassman has also been prominent in advocacy efforts on state and national levels for health system reform to improve oral health systems for a wide variety of underserved groups.

Michael Helgeson, D.D.S., is one of the founders of Apple Tree Dental, an innovative nonprofit organization that operates nine Centers for Dental Health and delivers onsite care in collaboration with more than 150 urban and rural organizations including Head Start Centers, schools, group homes, hospitals, medical clinics, and nursing facilities. In 2020, Apple Tree opened a Center for Dental Health within the Mayo Clinic Health System campus in Fairmont, Minnesota, and in 2023 it added the ADT Center for Dental Health in Minneapolis. He serves as Apple Tree's chief executive officer, managing a professional staff of more than 280, which delivered more than $44 million worth of dental care during 2023. Apple Tree's community collaborative practice model has been replicated in North Carolina, Louisiana, and California and has received recognition from the surgeon general, the American Dental Association, and the Robert Wood Johnson and Kellogg foundations. In 2017, he was included in a list of the 32 most influential people in dentistry published by *Incisal Edge*, and in 2019, the American Association for Community Dental Programs selected Helgeson for the John P. Rossetti Community Oral Health Impact Award in recognition of his leadership at the local, state, and national levels.

Helen Lee, M.D., M.P.H., is a tenured associate professor in the Department of Anesthesiology, with adjunct appointments in medical education and pediatric dentistry, University of Illinois Chicago. Lee is the director of the College of Medicine's Medical Scholars Program, which is a guaranteed B.A. to M.D. program with an undergraduate student body of approximately 145 students. As director, Lee manages a unique education curriculum designed to prepare an elite group of undergraduate students for a career in medicine.

Lee's research has focused on populations, outcomes, and factors that contribute to care at the intersection of medicine and dentistry. Prior work has relied on health services research methodology. Currently Lee and her co-principal investigator (PI), Dr. Joanna Buscemi, are developing and testing a behavioral intervention in a clinical trial. Lee is the co-PI of an NIH/

NIDCR (funding period 2022–2029) UG3/UH3 award (UG3DE032003), "Testing a Multibehavioral Intervention to Improve Oral Health Behaviors in the Pediatric Dental Surgery Population." Lee's work has been supported by the Foundation for Anesthesia Education and Research, UIC CCTS KL2, and the Department of Anesthesiology, University of Washington T32. Lee is board certified in anesthesiology and pediatric anesthesiology.

Kaz Rafia, D.D.S., M.B.A., M.P.H., serves as chief health equity officer, executive vice president of CareQuest Institute for Oral Health. In his role, he spearheads strategic initiatives to foster and advance engagement and access to integrated oral health care for the underserved and under-represented communities. Rafia also drives the organization's efforts to elevate the integration of oral health and overall health care through the oversight of the health improvement and grantmaking teams.

Rafia brings over 2 decades of experience in successful startups, academia, managed care, government, and nonprofit organizations. Prior to CareQuest Institute, Rafia served as the state dental director for the Oregon Health Authority, where he set the equity-centered State Oral Health Strategic Plan focusing on population health measures, health care workforce development, optimization of the value-based care coordination model, and telehealth. Previously, Rafia was the director of operations for the Partnership for International Medical Access–Northwest, building sustainable long-term international partnerships with culturally diverse authorities and leaders to better understand and serve their needs. Rafia was also a founding partner of Rafia Dental, a clinical associate professor at Oregon Health & Science University, and a clinic director at Kaiser Permanente. Rafia holds a doctor of dental surgery degree from the Ohio State University, a master of business administration degree from University of Illinois, and a master of public health degree from Johns Hopkins University.

Leah Stein Duker, Ph.D., OTR/L, is an occupational therapist and assistant professor in the Chan Division of Occupational Science and Occupational Therapy at the University of Southern California. Her research focuses on the broad-ranging effects of environmental factors on stress, well-being, and engagement during challenging health care encounters and the efficacy of tailored environmentally based interventions to alleviate these challenges. For the last 15 years, her work has explored the oral health challenges experienced by children with disabilities and their caregivers, as well as the benefits of adapting the environment to improve dental care for these populations (e.g., children with autism spectrum disorder).

Stein Duker is currently funded by a NIH/NIDCR UG3/UH3 grant to explore the efficacy of adapting the sensory environment of the dental office to decrease behavioral and physiological distress in children with and without dental fear and anxiety. Her research interests include autism, sensory processing, multisensory environments, and both traditional wired and innovative wireless techniques for measuring psychophysiological stress and anxiety. Her work has examined care in a variety of settings, including dentistry, primary care, oncology, emergency medicine, and mobile health (mHealth). In 2021, she was a recipient of the American Occupational Therapy Foundation's A. Jean Ayres Award for commitment to research-related development or testing of occupational therapy, especially in sensory processing.

Randi Tillman, D.M.D., M.B.A., is currently the executive dental director for the Health Care Services Corporation, which consists of the Blue Cross and Blue Shield plans for Illinois, Texas, Oklahoma, New Mexico, and Montana. Prior to this position, she spent 5 years as the chief dental officer at Guardian. She has a D.M.D. from the University of Pennsylvania and an M.B.A. from Columbia University. Tillman has more than 35 years of business experience in dental insurance, managed care, and health economics.

In addition to her career in the dental benefits industry, Tillman spent 10 years in the pharmaceutical and biotech industries, in health economics and outcomes research. In recent years, her focus has evolved to issues related to utilization management, wellness, and medical–dental integration. Tillman has served in multiple leadership positions over the course of her career. She served as a board member of the Gies Foundation for the Advancement of Dentistry for 7 years and was also the principal investigator for a grant from the National Institutes of Health, during her tenure as an associate professor at the Columbia University School of Dental and Oral Surgery. She has been a member of the American Association of Dental Consultants for over 20 years and is president-elect for 2024–2025.

Betsy Lee White, RDH, B.S., FSCDH, completed her A.A.S. degree in dental hygiene at Guilford Technical Community College in 1995 and her B.S. studies at the University of North Carolina School of Dentistry in 1997. She holds a fellowship in special care dentistry from the North Carolina Dental Hygiene Academy of Advanced Studies and a fellowship in special care dental hygiene from the Special Care Dentistry Association. Her commitment to special-care populations has been the center of her entire career. In 1994, White joined Dr. Bill Milner in his part-time practice and together created Access Dental Care. Access Dental Care has grown over 20-plus years and serves over 180 skilled nursing facilities, group homes for those with intellectual and developmental disabilities, Program of All-Inclusive Care for the Elderly (PACE) programs across the state of North Carolina, a regional HIV/AIDS program, and a community program for the older adults in New Hanover County.

White received the Sarah Bradshaw Award from Special Care Advocates in Dentistry, and she is the 2023 corecipient of the NC Council on Developmental Disabilities Holly Riddle Distinguished Service Award. She is currently serving on the NC Institute of Medicine, Medicaid Payment Transformation Committee; All Ages, All Stages NC Overall Health and Well-Being Taskforce; and Special Care Dentistry Association's Task Force on Dental Coverage in Medicare.

Appendix E

Members of the Global Forum on Innovation in Health Professional Education[1]

Jody Frost, PT, D.P.T., Ph.D., FAPTA, FNAP (Cochair)
Education Consultant and Facilitator

Zohray Talib, M.D. (Cochair)
Executive Vice Dean for Education and Professor of Medical Education and Medicine
California University of Science and Medicine, School of Medicine

Jonathan "Yoni" Amiel, M.D.
Interim Co-Vice Dean for Education
Senior Associate Dean for Curricular Affairs
Columbia Vagelos College of Physicians and Surgeons

Richard Berman, M.H.A, M.B.A.
Associate Vice President Strategic Initiatives
University of South Florida

Agnes Binagwaho, M.D., M.(Ped.), Ph.D.
Vice Chancellor and Professor of the Practice of Global Health Delivery
University of Global Health Equity

---

[1] The National Academies of Sciences, Engineering, and Medicine's forums and roundtables do not issue, review, or approve individual documents. The responsibility for the published Proceedings of a Workshop rests with the workshop rapporteurs and the institution.

Andrew P. Boucher
Chief Operating Officer/Interim Chief Executive Officer
National Register of Health Service

Anthony Breitbach, Ph.D., ATC, FASAHP, FNAP
Professor and Vice Dean
Saint Louis University

Reamer L. Bushardt, Pharm.D., PA-C, DFAAPA
Provost and Vice President for Academic Affairs
MGH Institute of Health Professions

Peter S. Cahn, Ph.D.
Associate Provost for Academic Affairs
MGH Institute of Health Professions

Robert Cain, D.O.
CEO
American Association of Colleges of Osteopathic Medicine

Kathy Chappell, Ph.D., R.N., FNAP, FAAN
Senior Vice President
Certification/Measurement, Accreditation, and Institute for Credentialing
    Research
American Nurses Credentialing Center

Steven Chesbro, PT, D.P.T., Ed.D.
Vice President for Education
American Physical Therapy Association

Mark Colip, O.D.
President
Association of Schools and Colleges of Optometry

Darrin D'Agostino, D.O., M.P.H., M.B.A.
Provost and Chief Academic Officer
Texas Tech University Health Sciences Center
American Association of Colleges of Osteopathic Medicine

Sanjay Desai, M.D.
Chief Academic Officer and Group Vice President of Medical Education
American Medical Association

Jan de Maeseneer, M.D., Ph.D., FRCGP (Hon.)
National Academy of Medicine Member
Department of Public Health and Primary Care,
Ghent University (Belgium)
Head WHO Collaborating Centre on Family Medicine and PHC—Ghent
University

Kylie P. Dotson-Blake, Ph.D., NCC, LPC
President and CEO
National Board for Certified Counselors, Inc., and Affiliates

Kim Dunleavy, Ph.D., MOMT, PT, OCS
Clinical Professor and Director of Community Engagement
University of Florida
American Council of Academic Physical Therapy

Kathrin (Katie) Eliot, Ph.D., R.D.
Director
Health Professions Educator
University of Oklahoma Health Sciences Center
Academy of Nutrition and Dietetics

Christopher Feddock, M.D., M.S., FAAP
Vice President of Competency-Based Assessment
National Board of Medical Examiners

Sara E. Fletcher, Ph.D.
Chief Executive Officer
Physician Assistant Education Association

Elizabeth (Liza) Goldblatt, Ph.D., M.P.A./H.A.
Director of National & Global Projects
Academy of Integrative Health and Medicine

Jennifer Graebe, M.S.N., NEA-BC
Director, Accreditation in Nursing Continuing Professional Development
and Joint Accreditation Programs
American Nurses Credentialing Center

Lynette Hamlin, Ph.D., R.N., CNM, FACNM
Professor and Associate Dean for Faculty Affairs
Uniformed Services University of Health Sciences

Kendra Harrington, PT, D.P.T., M.S.
Board-Certified Clinical Specialist in Women's Health Physical Therapy
Director, Residency/Fellowship Accreditation
American Board of Physical Therapy Residency and Fellowship Education
American Physical Therapy Association

Neil Harvison, Ph.D., OTR/L, FAOTA
Chief Academic and Scientific Affairs Officer
American Occupational Therapy Association

Eric Holmboe, M.D.
Chief Executive Officer
Intealth

Lisa Howley, M.Ed., Ph.D.
Senior Director of Strategic Initiatives and Partnerships
Association of American Medical Colleges

Cheryl L. Hoying, Ph.D., R.N., NEA-BC, FAONL, FACHE, FAAN
Chief Nurse Executive and Patient Care Services Officer
The Ohio State University Wexner Medical Center
National League for Nursing

Barry Issenberg, M.D.
President-Elect
Society for Simulation in Healthcare

Emilia Iwu, M.S.N., R.N., APNC, FWACN
Professor
Rutgers University

Pamela Jeffries, Ph.D., R.N., FAAN, ANEF
Dean of Nursing
Vanderbilt University

Nasreen Jessani, D.P.H, M.S.P.H.
Associate Faculty
Johns Hopkins Bloomberg School of Public Health
Faculty: Senior Researcher
Stellenbosch University

Kathryn (Kathy) Kolasa, Ph.D., RDN, LDN
Professor Emeritus and Master Educator, Department of Family Medicine—
Nutrition and Patient Education
East Carolina University Brody School of Medicine
Academy of Nutrition and Dietetics

Lyuba Konopasek, M.D.
Senior Associate Dean for Education
Quinnipiac University
Intealth

Kimberly Lomis, M.D.
Vice President, Medical Education Innovations
American Medical Association

Beverly Malone, Ph.D., R.N., FAAN
National Academy of Medicine Member
Chief Executive Officer
National League for Nursing

Dawn M. Mancuso, MAM, CAE, FASAE
Executive Director
Association of Schools and Colleges of Optometry

Rance McClain, D.O.
Senior Vice President of Medical Education
American Association of Colleges of Osteopathic Medicine

Karen McDonnell, Ph.D.
Associate Professor
Milken Institute School of Public Health
George Washington University

Lemmietta G. McNeilly, Ph.D., CCC-SLP, CAE
Chief Staff Officer, Speech-Language Pathology
ASHA Fellow
American Speech-Language-Hearing Association

Mark Merrick, Ph.D., ATC, FNATA
Professor and Dean
College of Health and Human Services
University of Toledo
Athletic Training Strategic Alliance

Warren Newton, M.D., M.P.H.
President and CEO
American Board of Family Medicine

Kate Brody Nooner, Ph.D., ABPP
Chair and Professor, Department of Psychology
University of North Carolina Wilmington
Adjunct Associate Professor, Department of Psychiatry and Behavioral
    Sciences
Duke University Medical Center
National Register of Health Service Psychologists

Loretta Nunez, M.A., Au.D., CCC-A/SLP, FNAP
Director of Academic Affairs and Research Education
ASHA Fellow
American Speech-Language-Hearing Association

David O'Bryon, J.D., CAE
President
Association of Chiropractic Colleges
Immediate-Past Chair
Academic Collaborative for Integrative Health

John Ogunkeye, M.S.
Executive Vice President
ACGME Global Services
Accreditation Council for Graduate Medical Education

Haru Okuda, M.D., FACEP, FSSH
Executive Director and CEO, USF Health CAMLS | HPCC
Associate Vice President, USF Health IPEP
Associate Dean Emerging Healthcare and Educational Technologies
Society for Simulation in Healthcare

Bjorg Palsdottir, M.P.A.
Executive Director and Cofounder
Training for Health Equity Network

Erin Patel, Psy.D., ABPP
Acting Chief of Health Professions Education
Veterans Health Administration

Stephanie Petrosky, D.C.N., M.H.A., RDN, LDN, FAND
Chair and Director, Department of Nutrition
Nova Southeastern University's College of Osteopathic Medicine

Andrea L. Pfeifle, Ed.D., PT, FNAP
Associate Vice President for Interprofessional Practice and Education
The Ohio State University and Wexner Medical Center
National Academies of Practice

Senthil Rajasekaran, M.D., MMHPE
Chief Academic Officer and Associate Dean, Academic Affairs at the
     Khalifa University
College of Medicine and Health Sciences in Abu Dhabi, United Arab
     Emirates

Sabrina Salvant, Ed.D., M.P.H., OTR/L
Director of Accreditation
American Occupational Therapy Association

Karen Sanders, M.D.
Deputy Chief Academic Affiliations Officer
U.S. Department of Veterans Affairs Office of Academic Affiliations

Joanne G. Schwartzberg, M.D.
Scholar-in-Residence
Accreditation Council for Graduate Medical Education

Wendi Schweiger, Ph.D., NCC, LPC
Director, NBCC International Capacity Building
Foundation and Professional Services
National Board for Certified Counselors, Inc., & Affiliates

Ryan Scilla, M.D., FACP, CPE
Associate Director, Medical and Dental Education
U.S. Department of Veterans Affairs Office of Academic Affiliations

Javaid I. Sheikh, M.D., M.B.A.
Dean
Weill Cornell Medicine—Qatar

Carl J. Sheperis, Ph.D.
Vice Provost and Dean of Graduate Studies
Kutztown University

Angela Simmons, Ph.D., RN, NEA-BC
Commandant, Associate Dean of Research
Uniformed Services University Graduate School of Nursing

Nancy Spector, Ph.D., RN
Director of Nursing Education
National Council of State Boards of Nursing

Jeffrey Stewart, D.D.S, M.S.
Senior Vice President for Interprofessional and Global Collaboration
American Dental Education Association

Melissa Trego, D.O., Ph.D.
Dean
Salus University, Pennsylvania College of Optometry
Association of Schools and Colleges of Optometry

Carole Tucker, Ph.D., M.S.
Associate Dean for Research
University of Texas–Galveston
American Council of Academic Physical Therapy

Haleavalu F. Ofahengaue Vakalahi, M.S.W., Ph.D.
President and CEO
Council on Social Work Education

Karen P. West, D.M.D., M.P.H.
President and CEO
American Dental Education Association

Alison J. Whelan, M.D.
Chief Medical Education Officer
Association of American Medical Colleges

GLOBAL FORUM STAFF

Patricia Cuff, M.P.H., M.S.
Forum Director and Senior Program Officer
Board on Global Health

Erika Chow
Research Assistant
Board on Global Health

Julie Pavlin, M.D., Ph.D., M.P.H.
Senior Director
Board on Global Health